Problems in Paediatrics

Problems in Practice Series

Problems in Practice Series

Series Editors : J.Fry K.G.D.Williams M.Lancaster-Smith

Problems
in
Paediatrics

John Hood
MRCP, MRCS

Consultant Paediatrician
Queen Mary's Hospital
Sidcup, Kent

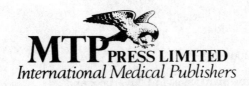

MTP PRESS LIMITED
International Medical Publishers

Published by
MTP Press Limited
Falcon House
Lancaster, England

First published 1982

British Library Cataloguing in Publication Data

Hood, John
    Problems in paediatrics.—(Problems in
    practice series)
    1. Pediatrics
    I. Title   II. Series
    618.92   RJ45

ISBN 0-85200-263-7

Typesetting by Swiftpages Ltd, Liverpool and
printed by Butler & Tanner Ltd,
Frome and London

Contents

Contents

cleft palate and tongue tie – Swellings in the neck – Ear, nose and throat surgery – The eyes – Neurosurgical conditions – Orthopaedic problems

Respiratory emergencies – Cardiac emergencies – Fits and coma – Metabolic emergencies – Gastro-intestinal emergencies – Genito-urinary emergencies – Miscellaneous emergencies

Preface

This book has been written with general practitioners primarily in view, describing common paediatric conditions that present in the outpatient clinics and those that require admission to hospital. The book is neither a textbook of paediatrics nor a handbook but is aimed to provide guidelines for the more commonplace conditions. Some aspects therefore, have been dealt with in detail, where felt relevant, while others are omitted on grounds of probable rare encounter. It is hoped that this volume will provide the family practitioner with an insight in the paediatrician's approach to many of the common problems in children and to help him decide on the best course of action to follow.

The care of children constitutes a significant and important part of a family doctor's work and practitioners are keen to promote optional care in all circumstances. It is hoped that the endeavours of this book will go in some small way to help put across the practitioner's approach.

John Hood

Series Foreword

This series of books is designed to help general practitioners. So are other books. What is unusual in this instance is their collective authorship; they are written by specialists working at district general hospitals. The writers derive their own experience from a range of cases less highly selected than those on which textbooks are traditionally based. They are also in a good position to pick out topics which they see creating difficulties for the practitioners of their district, whose personal capacities are familiar to them; and to concentrate on contexts where mistakes are most likely to occur. They are all well-accustomed to working in consultation.

All the authors write from hospital experience and from the viewpoint of their specialty. There are, therefore, matters important to family practice which should be sought not within this series, but elsewhere. Within the series much practical and useful advice is to be found with which the general practitioner can compare his existing performance and build in new ideas and improved techniques.

These books are attractively produced and I recommend them.

J. P. Horder OBE
President, The Royal College
of General Practitioners

1 Infant feeding

*Breast feeding – Bottle feeding – Vitamins – Regurgitation –
Vomiting – Colic – The hungry baby – The baby who does not
feed*

Patterns of feeding babies vary worldwide and have varied in
the Western world from decade to decade. The past 50 years
have seen the pendulum swing from breast feeding to almost
entire bottle feeding but the past decade has seen renewed
enthusiasm for breast feeding which, in part, has been due to
medical evidence demonstrating more clearly its advantages,
the rising cost of formula feeds and fashion.

Breast feeding

This is accepted as the first choice in feeding of babies in the
first 6 months of life even though most present day well-known
milk formulae have been significantly improved. These benefits
are shown in Table 1.1.

Early education of mother
    Education of the mother during pregnancy, especially con-
cerning infant feeding, is most important. Those mothers who
discuss this with their midwife or doctor in early pregnancy and
decide to breast feed are far more likely to succeed in feeding
their baby and will sustain lactation for a longer time than those
who are persuaded to feed at the time of delivery. Education
should be taken, ideally, into the school classroom so that young
adolescents of both sexes have some idea of the important

Care of breasts
aspects of child rearing. Antenatal advice concerning care of
the breasts is important, particularly in relation to inverted

13

Table 1.1   Advantages of breast feeding

Mother	Baby
1. Time in preparing feeds eliminated. Saves cost of formula feeds.	1. Significant reduction in risk from infection: (a) eliminates risk of contamination and wrongly prepared feed (b) phagocytosis of bacteria by cells in maternal milk (c) secretory IgA giving protection against pathogenic *E. coli* infection and some viruses (d) lactoferrin which inhibits growth of pathogenic coliforms.
2. Benefits to maternal health. Some reduction in tendency to gain weight after pregnancy. Reduced risk of breast carcinoma in later life.	
3. Superior bonding between mother and baby, usually enhancing the normal enjoyment of motherhood. Non-accidental injury (NAI) a rare occurrence among mothers who breast feed.	2. Affords some protection against allergic disorders. 3. Superior bonding between mother and baby.

Early suckling

nipples and those with delicate skin who may be prone to cracked nipples in the postnatal period. At delivery it is a great advantage to put the baby to the breast immediately as this is a vital step in bonding and establishing lactation. In the first 3 days it is important to realise that the initial volumes of milk produced are small and that the quality (the constituents of the colostrum) counts for more than the volume of feed. Secondly, most babies are not avid feeders in the first few days of life and in the full term baby of normal birth-weight no detriment will be suffered from only a modest intake during the first few days of life. It is vital in the immediate postnatal period that mothers

Importance of reassurance

are given good advice and reassurance from the midwifery and medical staff concerning feeding, otherwise they may lose confidence in their ability to feed their baby and decide at an early stage to change to bottle feeding. A sequence of events is shown in Table 1.2.

Mothers who are unable to breast feed

While most mothers will establish breast feeding without too much difficulty, there are those who fail to lactate adequately, those with severely inverted nipples and those who, for medical and obstetric reasons, are unable to establish lactation. It is very important under these circumstances to be very reassuring to the mother and not to let her in any way feel inadequate from failing to breast feed her baby because of circumstances beyond her control. Explanation of the advantages and disadvantages of breast and bottle feeding should be carefully

Table 1.2 Patterns of events in first week

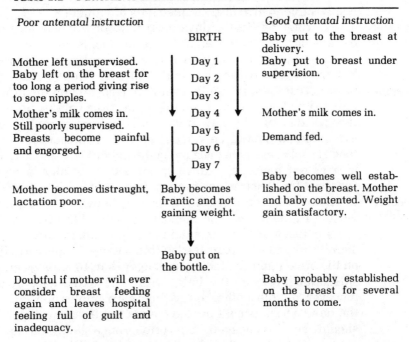

Poor antenatal instruction		Good antenatal instruction
	BIRTH	Baby put to the breast at delivery.
Mother left unsupervised.	Day 1	Baby put to breast under supervision.
Baby left on the breast for too long a period giving rise to sore nipples.	Day 2	
	Day 3	
Mother's milk comes in.	Day 4	Mother's milk comes in.
Still poorly supervised.	Day 5	Demand fed.
Breasts become painful and engorged.	Day 6	
	Day 7	
		Baby becomes well established on the breast. Mother and baby contented. Weight gain satisfactory.
Mother becomes distraught, lactation poor.	Baby becomes frantic and not gaining weight.	
	Baby put on the bottle.	
Doubtful if mother will ever consider breast feeding again and leaves hospital feeling full of guilt and inadequacy.		Baby probably established on the breast for several months to come.

explained to mothers in the ante-natal period and although it is medically accepted that breast feeding is predominantly the best mode of feeding newborn babies, it must always be remembered that it is the duty of medical personnel to advise and not tell mothers, since the ultimate choice is emphatically theirs. Time spent instructing primigravida mothers is the most important of all since, after successfully breast feeding their first baby, most will continue to breast feed subsequent off-spring. On the whole most mothers who have bottle fed their babies from previous pregnancies will continue to do so, although a small percentage do decide to change, often having been shy to assert their preference in the days when the bottle prevailed.

Primigravida mothers

There are few contra-indications to breast feeding. Severe debilitating illnesses of the mother are a main contra-indication but less severe illnesses including urinary tract infections, breast abscesses, are not. Medication given to the mother does appear in the breast milk but seldom in sufficient quantity to produce any ill-effect to the baby. Exceptions include antineoplastic drugs, antithyroid drugs, radiopharmaceuticals, amantadine and lithium carbonate. Babies can be continued to be

Contra-indications to breast feeding

breast fed by mothers on anticoagulants (warfarin sodium) but it is advisable to give oral supplements of vitamin K.

Early weight trends

During the first 4 days most newborn babies lose up to 6–10% of their body weight. Once feeding is well established there is a steady weight gain of 15–20 g per day and often more. Failure to gain weight is usually an indication of inadequate intake.

Test feeding

Test feeding can be useful in ascertaining the intake of milk but it should be realized that it has little validity until after the 6th day of life and that a full 24 hour period must be evaluated. It should be remembered that indiscriminate test feeding only serves to promote maternal anxiety which in itself is a potent cause of failure to lactate, so it should only be reserved for absolute necessities. Demand feeding is preferred

Feeding schedules

to 4 hourly feeding except for the sleepy baby who requires to be woken 4 hourly and the small baby who, likewise, requires regular feeds until he is gaining weight satisfactorily. Babies usually take most of their feed within the first 5 minutes of fixing on the breast and so feeding for longer than 10 minutes on each side often provides the baby with little extra milk. It does, however, put the mother at risk from sore nipples and so putting the baby on the breast for too long in the first few days of life should be discouraged, but often, once lactation is fully established, the mother's nipples acclimatize to the baby sucking and then little harm can be done from leaving the baby on for longer periods. Overall the more vigorously and frequently the baby sucks, the more the mother will lactate and vice versa. For the baby who is slow in gaining weight, it is therefore profitable to put the baby to the breast more frequently, rather than to leave the baby on the breast for longer periods which is often done to no avail.

Clinic checks on weight gain

Clinic checks are important to check the baby's weight gain is within reasonable expectation. The usual weight gain in the first 3 months is 20–30 g per day and after 3 months 15 g per day and most babies double their birth weight by 5 months and treble it by one year. Percentile charts are useful in charting a baby's progress during the first year of life so that the overall trend can be seen at a glance. Mothers should not be panicked by a slight deviation from the norm, providing the baby is otherwise healthy. It should be remembered that with breast fed babies there can be a situation where, after being breast fed for up to 2–4 months, maternal lactation can fall off but the baby still remains contented but does not gain weight. Obesity in breast fed babies can occur but unless there is familial obesity many of these babies slim down after the first year of life.

Curtailing feeding is usually seldom necessary unless the mother has such a glut of milk that the baby tends to regurgitate and have loose motions, in which case some limitation of intake is desirable.

Formula feed complements

Complementing feeding with formula feed on occasions is required when there is sustained inadequacy of maternal lactation but complementing of breast feeding otherwise only detracts from the benefits of such feeding in the first place.

Breast feeding is stopped all too often after discharge home and the reasons for this include 'my milk was not strong enough', 'the baby vomited', 'the baby had runny stools' or 'I had to go on antibiotics'. None of these are, of course, valid but the mother who is uncertain will often decide to change because she thinks it is the safest move in the absence of adequate reassurance.

Bottle feeding

Although there has been a substantial trend towards breast feeding, many babies are still bottle fed and many of those who are initially breast fed later become bottle fed babies for one

Table 1.3 Composition of various milks

	Breast milk	Cow's milk	SMA Gold Cap	Osterfeed	Cow & Gate Premium
Energy (cal/100 ml)	70	65	65	68	65
Protein (g/100 ml)	1.34	3.5	1.56	1.45	1.83
% Casein	40	71	40	39	33
% Whey	60	23	60	61	67
Carbohydrate (g/100 ml)	7.0	4.5	7.2	7.0	6.9
Fat (g/100 ml)	4.2	4.4	3.6	3.8	3.4
Sodium (mg/100 ml)	15	22	15	19	22
Calcium (mg/100 ml)	35	117	44	36	48
Phosphorus (mg/100 ml)	15	92	33	31	31
Iron (mg/100 ml)	76	50	1,270	960	650

Cow's milk

reason or another. Raw cow's milk itself is a totally unsuitable food for babies during the first 6 months of life but most of the current milk formulae have been adapted to remove the main hazards of cow's milk and to provide the baby with a satisfactory calorie intake. The compositions of breast milk as compared to cow's milk and some of the currently available milk formulae is shown in Table 1.3.

Energy and fluid requirements

In bottle feeding it is important to be able to calculate the baby's energy and fluid intake. The full-term baby requires 50–55 kcal/lb/day or 110–120 kcal/kg/day. The child of 1 year requires 45 kcal/lb/day or 100 kg/day. With regard to fluids the full-term baby requires 2–3 ozs/lb/day or 130–190 ml/kg/day. In imperial measurements 1 oz of milk yields 20 kcal. A baby requires 2.5 oz (50 kcal)/lb/day. In metric measurement 100 mls of milk yields 67 kcal. A baby requires 150–160 ml (110 kcal)/kg/day. It should always be emphasized that feeds are calculated on the expected weight of the baby and not on the actual body weight (unless they coincide).

Weaning

Weaning should commence at about 4–5 months or when the baby weighs more than 5 kg. Babies will, of course, take weaning diet a lot earlier but this does give a high solute load and incurs the risk of hyperosmolar dehydration. The guidelines cannot be absolute but because of the hyperosmolar risk, it is better to advise later weaning than earlier.

Vitamins

Vitamin K

Vitamin K should be given at birth to all babies who have had a traumatic delivery. It should also be given to all newborns undergoing surgery and those who are on intravenous fluids or only receiving clear fluids orally for any sustained period. Babies who are breast fed and those that are pre-term likewise should receive vitamin K. Dosage is phytomenadione (vitamin K_1) 1.0 mg, i.m. for babies 2.0 kg and over and 0.5 mg for babies less than 2.0 kg. Oral vitamin K, 1.0 mg on alternate days can be given orally for those babies who are breast fed and whose mothers are receiving warfarin (or other coumarin or indandione preparations). It is not necessary for those mothers receiving heparin only. The recommended dosage should not be exceeded except in cases of proven haemorrhagic disease of the newborn since, otherwise, it can precipitate hyperbilirubinaemia.

Other vitamins

Vitamins are required for normal health and growth. The daily requirements for babies are as follows:

Vitamin A	1 400 iu (international units)	
Vitamin D	400 iu (800 iu for premature babies)	
Vitamin C	35.0 mg	
Vitamin B	thiamine, B_1	0.3 mg
	riboflavine, B_2	0.4 mg
	pyridoxine, B_6	0.3 mg
	nicotinamide, B_7	5.0 mg
	vitamin B_{12}	0.3 mg
Vitamin E	tocopherol	4.0 mg

Vitamin D

The common milk formulae have vitamin supplements which are entirely sufficient for the full term baby. Pre-term babies, especially those under 2.5 kg in weight, should receive additional supplements during the first year of life. Breast fed babies should also receive vitamin supplements after the first month of life, as the vitamin D content may be low and this is particularly important for the coloured baby reared in this country with relatively low exposure to sunlight. Excessive vitamin D should not be given (not exceeding 400 iu daily in the full term baby) as this will give rise to hypervitaminosis D with resultant hypercalcaemia and nephrocalcinosis.

Regurgitation

Persistent regurgitation

It is normal for babies to bring back some feed after winding and providing that the baby is otherwise healthy and gaining weight there is no need for concern. Some babies will persistently regurgitate between feeds as well but much of the vomitus contains clear fluid as well as milk and this is often a source of distress to parents because they fear that the baby may not be retaining sufficient feed and, in addition, there is also a smell of vomitus not only on the baby's clothes but very often on the parents as well. Provided the baby is otherwise healthy and gaining weight, it is important to reassure the parents stating that the condition is self-limiting and will largely resolve by the age of one year. It is probably due to a combination of impaired gastro-oesophageal sphincter control coupled with a fluid diet and being predominantly in a horizontal posture. As time progresses the cardia becomes more competent, the baby is eating more solid food and is then in an erect posture, from which time the problem rapidly resolves. There are some babies

'Ruminators'

who are ruminators and they induce vomiting by putting their fingers down their throat and this has to be looked for and, if necessary, mittens applied to prevent the habit.

19

Failure to
thrive

In circumstances where persistent vomiting does occur and the baby is not thriving and full examination has excluded all other causes, Nestargel (methylcellulose) can be used to thicken the feeds and in most instances it is very effective. While in many babies there is no obvious cause for their regurgitation, in all probability the technique of feeding and over-feeding are the background factors.

Vomiting

Vomiting, particularly in association with failure to gain weight or a baby that is unwell, requires immediate investigation. Among some of the causes include congenital hypertrophic pyloric stenosis and other congenital anomalies of the gastro-intestinal tract, gastroenteritis, septicaemia, meningitis, raised intracranial pressure and adrenal cortex dysfunction.

Colic

Symptoms

This is frequent in the 2–4 month period. The symptoms are of a baby who screams incessantly during and after a feed. The baby is flushed and agitated and usually kicks and draws up his legs. There are many possible causes of colic but often the cause is either not obvious or is unknown. The baby who is difficult to wind may well be prone to colic. Maternal anxiety is often mani-fested by a restless and crying baby, although in all fairness, this, in most instances, is secondary to the baby's original problem. Serious consideration has to be given to the possibility of intussusception if the baby looks ill and pale between scream-ing attacks or passes blood rectally. This is usually a condition that occurs towards the end of the first year of life rather than in the first few weeks. Occasionally fits in infancy present as apparent colic with some screaming attacks and for this reason it is important to witness an actual attack to see how a baby behaves. Cow's milk protein intolerance is known to produce colic as well as other food intolerances.

Possibility of
intus-
susception

Anti-
spasmodics

For those babies for whom there is no obvious cause anti-spasmodics (e.g. Dicyclomine 0.5 mg/kg) given 20 minutes before feeds often alleviates the symptoms.

The hungry baby

Some babies demand more food than they apparently need. The pre-term and particularly the small-for-dates babies during a period of catch-up growth will often feed ravenously and this is of course to their benefit. In the full term baby who is already thriving satisfactorily, it is important to see that the parents are not interpreting all reactions of the baby as due to hunger since often picking the baby up and cuddling him or changing a dirty nappy will pacify him as much as giving a further feed. It should be remembered that there are wide variations in the feeding requirements of babies and providing that the feeding regime is not ridiculously inappropriate, the situation is probably best left since the baby will probably, in the course of time, level out to fairly normal food intake. Although weaning diet is not usually recommended until after 4 months of age, there are some babies who are ravenously hungry, where introduction of weaning diet at an earlier stage can be justified providing this is not excessive.

Excess weight gain

Although wide variations in feeding occur, excess weight gain to the degree of obesity is not always desirable. Those babies whose parents are non-obese usually slim down as they get older, while in those of obese parents this may be a progressive tendency. In such circumstances advice on excess feeding is obviously important.

The baby who does not feed

These babies do cause concern, particularly if they are significantly under-weight and if this is part of a pattern of general failure to thrive, obviously this needs full investigation. There are babies, however, who are reluctant feeders who appear fit and well but gain weight consistently along the lower centiles. Very often this is a familial or even racial trend and providing the child is otherwise healthy and their growth velocity and stature is normal, it is important to avoid producing anxiety in their parents' mind because they are not in the upper centiles of weight gain.

All problems in feeding should be regarded in context of the infant's health and overall progress and wide variation will occur in infant feeding patterns in spite of medical advice and in many instances it is a matter of 'who are we to criticize'.

2 Respiratory diseases

UPPER RESPIRATORY TRACT INFECTION

Tonsillitis – Otitis media – Stridor – Croup – Acute epiglottitis

Susceptibility of young children This is extremely common in young children and many younger children get up to six or more such infections a year. All ages are vulnerable but there are certain peaks of incidence at different ages as well as seasonal variance. The toddler beginning to socialize with older children is readily susceptible, as is the child who is just beginning school. Some children, like adults, are more vulnerable to infection than others and social circumstances also play a part, including overcrowding, smoking habits in the household and stress. Many parents seek advice thinking that something is wrong with their child and wanting advice on prevention. It is possible that such pressures bend some doctors into prolific prescription of antibiotics which, in fact, are seldom indicated.

Respiratory tract infections in babies Babies are the most susceptible to upper respiratory tract infections. Breast feeding does afford some protection in the early weeks but all the same, many acquire infection. Blockage of the nasal airway gives rise to the main difficulty and it should be realized that babies in the first 6 months of life are obligatory nasal breathers and thus with a blocked nasal airway they are unable to feed. The essential measure is to keep the nasal airway clear, wiping the nose and if necessary, to irrigate with saline nasal drops before feeds. The use of ephedrine 0.5% in saline or similar decongestant nasal drops are seldom indicated. Many upper respiratory tract infections are accompanied by a cough but usually this does not require any specific

23

treatment. Linctus simplex can be prescribed for symptomatic
relief but cough suppressants and allied medications are of little
objective effect. Overall, medication for an upper respiratory
tract infection is best avoided, except for relief of troublesome
symptoms.

Persistent
rhinorrhoea

There are some children who have persistent rhinorrhoea
– the so-called 'catarrhal child'. It should be remembered that
some of these suffer from perennial allergic rhinitis rather than
the recurrent infection. Rarely, persistent rhinorrhoea may be
due to choanal stenosis and so the nasal airway should be
checked by passing a nasal catheter to see if it is patent. Foreign
bodies likewise produce recurrent nasal discharge and blocked
nasal airway which should be apparent from the history and
examination. Many children with chronic rhinitis have concurrent adenoidal hypertrophy and as an initial measure, a
nasal decongestant such as Actifed or Dimotapp is often helpful.
If the nasal obstruction is persistent in the presence of
adenoidal hypertrophy, then removal of the adenoids may be
advisable.

Tonsillitis

This is often over-diagnosed, especially by parents. The
pharynx, in an upper respiratory tract infection is red and
congested but in tonsillitis the tonsils are specifically inflamed,
swollen and exude pus. Although many tonsillar infections are
due to viruses, including the Epstein–Barr virus, causing infectious mononucleosis, others can be due to bacterial infections
which include beta-haemolytic streptococcus. If there is a likelihood of bacterial infection penicillin is still probably the most
effective antibiotic. For the very ill child it is reasonable to give
the first dose by injection and complete the rest of the course
orally.

Otitis media

This is a common infection in children as this is in part related to
their susceptibility to upper respiratory tract infections and due
to the fact that the Eustachian tube is shorter and infection more
easily spreads to the middle ear. Many children will have
otalgia with minor respiratory tract infections and on examination there is slight pinkness of the periphery of the drum. Many
parents say their children have had discharging ears when, in
fact, it has only been normal loss of soft wax from the external

Symptoms auditory meatus. The symptoms of otitis media in children are usually pain and crying and the older child will complain of earache but the infant may well cry incessantly and the toddler may complain of abdominal pain. Otoscopic examination of the tympanic membrane shows an intensive red and congested drum with a loss of the normal right reflex. Pus may later be seen behind the membrane and later there may be evidence of perforation. Many children with a mild upper respiratory tract infection have slight pinkness of the periphery of the eardrum and, likewise, screaming babies may also have some pinkness. This dose not constitute genuine otitis media and does not require treatment as such.

Treatment

Perforation of ear drum
While many cases are related to a viral upper respiratory tract infection, middle ear infection may also be caused by bacterial infection such as *Haemophilus influenzae* and *Strep. pneumoniae*. Penicillin is effective for otitis media and ampicillin can also be used. If the drum is perforated gentamicin and hydrocortisone ear drops are quite helpful in irrigating the exterior auditory canal and treating a concurrent otitis externa. For the child who has chronic rhinorrhea, a nasal decongestant might well help to reduce recurrent attacks of otitis media and, likewise, if there is significant adenoidal hypertrophy, removal of the adenoids may well be beneficial.

Stridor

Double aortic arch
Many newborn babies have an inspiratory stridor due to a floppy epiglottis. The baby is otherwise healthy and has no distress. As the child grows older, the airway becomes bigger and the condition spontaneously resolves. For those who have persisting stridor beyond the age of 6 months, this might be due to extrinsic pressure and one such cause is a double aortic arch, which also compresses the oesophagus and may cause vomiting. A barium swallow with a lateral view often shows indentation of the posterior aspect of the upper third of the oesophagus. The condition is amenable to vascular surgery.

Croup

This is a condition peculiar to children between the ages of 6 months and 3 years. Simple croup occurs in toddlers and usually commences quite abruptly later in the evening when the child has just gone to bed. There is a hacking cough associated with a marked inspiratory stridor. There is usually only slight fever and no other malaise. When the condition is mild there are no signs of respiratory distress such as intercostal recession, sternal retraction, supraclavicular indrawing or tracheal tug. Usually if the child can be coaxed back to sleep the condition resolves within 24 hours. The causative organism is thought to be the para influenza virus.

Treatment

Sudden
airway
obstruction

Moisturised air and mild sedation are usually effective. Antibiotics are not indicated. Although the illness is usually mild and benign, it does require careful surveillance because there are some children who develop, quite suddenly, severe airway obstruction, often needing intubation or tracheostomy.

Acute epiglottitis

Course of
illness

This is a potentially fatal condition unless immediate action is taken. The onset is usually of abrupt inspiratory stridor with cough, fever and general malaise. The age range is much wider than for those children with croup and the course of the illness is far more rapid and severe with increasing airway obstruction. Prompt admission to hospital is required as the child may require intubation or tracheostomy. An extremely ill child may not struggle for breath but instead will look grey, and sweaty and cyanosed. The child requires immediate intubation since he is at a point of impending respiratory arrest.

It is inadvisable in these children to do anything that could induce gagging and laryngeal spasm. On examination only the anterior third of the tongue can be depressed carefully and a large cherry-red mound may be seen arising from the larynx due to a grossly oedematous epiglottis.

Cause

The causal organism is usually a type B *Haemophilus influenzae* which is often isolated from blood culture. The child

Treatment

should have high doses of ampicillin or chloramphenicol to eradicate this organism.

It is essential to get the child to hospital as quickly as possible, forwarning the staff that intubation or tracheostomy may be necessary. 100 mg of hydrocortisone given intravenously can sometimes reduce the oedema sufficiently until an

Intubation

airway can be inserted. A nasoendotracheal tube inserted for

48–72 hours suffices until the oedema resolves. Tracheostomy may be required but this is less commonly indicated than previously. Should a child have complete airway obstruction prior to transfer to hospital, insertion of a large syringe needle through the cricothyroid membrane may be lifesaving.

Risk of infection

It has been shown that other children in close proximity to children that have had acute epiglottis are susceptible and so it is important to observe the family carefully, as well as notify play groups and schools.

CHEST INFECTIONS

Pneumonias – Lobar pneumonia – Airways obstruction – Asthma

Bronchitis

Bronchitis can complicate upper respiratory tract infections as part of a descending respiratory tract infection. The clinical features are fever, cough and mild dyspnoea. Unlike in adults, it is more commonly of viral origin, so antibiotics are usually of no benefit. Simple supportive treatment is usually effective. Linctus simplex can help a troublesome cough but other cough suppressants are usually best avoided except possibly at night if the cough is unproductive.

Pneumonias

Bronchopneumonia is more common in young children. It may be either viral or bacterial in origin. It often complicates common infectious illnesses of children such as measles, pertussis and chickenpox.

Treatment

Treatment logically depends on aetiology and may be difficult to establish. Bacterial pneumonias indicate the use of antibiotics whereas viral pneumonias show little response. Since the number of organisms isolated in such instances is low, it is often necessary to start antibiotics in any case particularly if the child is sick. Penicillin, started initially by an intramuscular injection, is effective and erythromycin and ampicillin can also be used. Expensive broad spectrum antibiotics do not show any particular benefit and are only likely to produce resistant organisms.

27

Lobar pneumonia

This is uncommon in toddlers and occurs more often in older
children. The causative organism is usually a *Pneumococcus*,
although other organisms including *Streptococcus, Staphylo-
coccus* and *Haemophilus influenzae* may occur. Penicillin is
usually the antibiotic of choice, initially given by intramuscular
injection if the child is sick. Physiotherapy is helpful if there
is extensive consolidation, although many children, once active,
require little help in this respect. While clinical signs are
important guidelines as to progress, it is often helpful when the
child is substantially recovering to obtain a chest X-ray to see
that the chest is radiologically clear because at times there can
be persisting consolidation when, in fact, there is little to be
heard through the stethoscope.

Causes

Treatment

X-ray

Possible
underlying
causes

It is to be remembered:

(1) The child with persistent collapse of the right lower lobe
    may have had an inhaled foreign body.
(2) If there is persistent right middle lobe collapse, this might
    be due to hilar adenopathy due to primary tuberculous
    infection.
(3) The child with recurrent chest infections may have cystic
    fibrosis.

Airways obstruction

Many children with respiratory tract infections develop
airways obstruction. Those children who have bronchitis may
have a wheeze due to oedema of the bronchioles and some of
these children may, later, become definitely asthmatic.

Symptoms

Acute bronchiolitis in infancy causes significant airway
obstruction. The illness is usually peculiar to infants between 2
months and 1 year of age. It starts with an upper respiratory
tract infection and after 48 hours the baby begins to wheeze and
has a persistent dry cough. The chest is found to be hyperinflated and on auscultation there are high-pitched inspiratory
and expiratory rhonchi. The baby may find it difficult to feed
because of the effect in breathing. This illness is caused by the
respiratory syncitial virus and tends to occur spasmodically
during the winter months.

Treatment

Treatment is supportive with moisture and some sedation
for the mild case and, because of the difficulty of feeding, half
strength feeds and more frequent feeds are helpful. The baby
with mild bronchiolitis can be nursed at home but if the airways

Hospital admission

obstruction is obviously increasing, admission to hospital will be necessary in case oxygen and intense humidification are required. Antibiotics are seldom helpful in this condition. A small dose of salbutamol may relieve their airways obstruction, although there is limited effect under the age of 18 months.

Asthma

Symptoms and signs

Constitutes a high proportion of out-patient and in-patient referrals. Some cases have a history of preceding atopy and, not infrequently, asthma follows infantile eczema. In many instances there is a family history of atopy. The symptoms usually begin between 2 and 3 years of age and the initial attacks are often ascribed to bronchitis with wheezing and there is a persistent recurrent cough. Many episodes are preceded by rhinorrhoea and sneezing, attributed to coryza but, in fact, probably due to allergic rhinitis. The clinical signs are typical with dyspnoea, often audible wheeze and on auscultation there are high-pitched expiratory rhonchi in both lung fields.

Discussion with family

Treatment firstly involves careful discussion with the family to explain the nature of asthma and the common influencing factors including allergy, infection, emotion and exercise. It is important to explain the mode of action of the prescribed medication so that the parents and child can use this intelligently. Reassurance is important to state that children seldom die from asthmatic attacks and the nature of the condition is such that it usually improves with age.

Broncho-dilators

In simple asthma, bronchodilators such as salbutamol are effective and given for attacks as they arise. It is best given at the initial onset of symptoms and for this reason it is a good idea to give the mother a good supply of it so that it can be started immediately without delay. There are some children who do not respond to oral salbutamol but may respond to the inhaled powder. For the child with recurrent asthma who is not controlled by simple measures, disodium cromoglycate is often helpful (Intal). It is important to stress to the child and to the parents that this is a prophylactic treatment and must be continued on a longterm basis for any benefit and that it is not helpful in an acute attack. Secondly it is important to train the child so that he uses the Intal effectively and also to see that the child is able to get his dosage when he is at school. Problems in medication arise in the child under 5 years. There are now a number of small portable pumps on the market which can be

Disodium cromoglycate

used to give nebulized salbutamol and disodium cromoglycate suspension by a face mask.

Long acting theophylline compounds have been used and some children find these beneficial.

In spite of bronchodilators and disodium cromoglycate, there are still some children who have recurrent severe asthma with persistent airways obstruction, associated with poor respiratory function and chronically hyperinflated chests. For these children it is reasonable to give a steroid inhaler, provided that the correct dosage is used. Its absorption through the lung surface is minimal and the likelihood of producing a Cushingoid affect slight.

Steroid inhaler

Children should not be put on to systemic steroids for asthma on a longterm basis unless there are compelling reasons. There is a definite place for the use of steroids in status asthmaticus but their longterm use is to be strongly resisted. This is because not only does it produce the side-effects well known in adults, but in addition they produce growth retardation. For those children with very severe asthma for whom there is no alternative, systemic steroids are given on an alternate day basis for the shortest time possible.

Risks of longterm steroids

In asthma, it is important to remember that many problems are set off by allergic causes. This may be elicited in the case history and skin tests are sometimes useful. Many asthmatics are sensitive to house dust and the house mite (*Dermatophygoides pteronyssinus*) and for this reason it is important to take procedures to minimize the house mite in the bedroom, including regularly vacuuming and damp dusting, cleaning and putting the mattress in a cover, using cotton mesh rather than wool blankets and manmade fibre duvets and pillows rather than feather ones. These measures help reduce the house mite population in the bedroom but of course they are never entirely eradicated.

Allergic causes

Desensitization is often mentioned by parents, but is seldom indicated as in atopic children it is not without its risks.

Desensitiz-ation

Infection

There are some children where asthma is precipitated by infection and if there is significant bronchitis, antibiotics are indicated. In many instances the so-called infection is due to concurrent allergic rhinitis.

Allergic Factors

Stress is well known to produce asthma and family tensions and problems at school have to be taken into account. For those children with a profound problem the Child Guidance Clinic may be helpful.

Implications of overall management

Over recent years there have been many useful additions to the therapeutics of asthma. It is therefore important to keep the treatment as simple and effective as possible. Due to the many medicines, there is a dangerous tendency to over-prescribe when, in fact, one medicine would be effective. Compliance to medication is directly related to simplicity. The aim is to keep the child well and at school. These days there is no need to send a child to a special school because of asthma.

Tendency to over-prescribe

Table 2.1 Common disorders of the respiratory tract

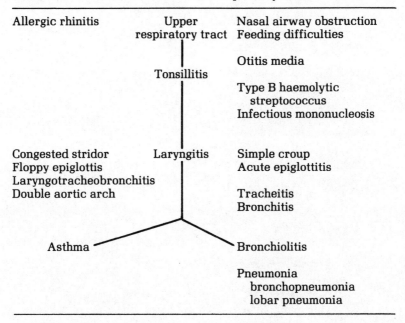

Allergic rhinitis	Upper respiratory tract	Nasal airway obstruction Feeding difficulties
	Tonsillitis	Otitis media
		Type B haemolytic streptococcus Infectious mononucleosis
Congested stridor Floppy epiglottis Laryngotracheobronchitis Double aortic arch	Laryngitis	Simple croup Acute epiglottitis
		Tracheitis Bronchitis
Asthma		Bronchiolitis
		Pneumonia bronchopneumonia lobar pneumonia

③ Gastro-intestinal problems

Gastro-enteritis and related problems – Malabsorption – Chronic inflammatory bowel disease – Congenital abnormalities – Large bowel obstruction – Appendicitis – Differential diagnosis

GASTRO-ENTERITIS AND RELATED PROBLEMS

This is still one of the more common infections in children and in infancy can be life-threatening and its dangers, therefore, should not be ignored.

Diarrhoea with vomiting

It should be remembered that gastroenteritis is *diarrhoea with vomiting*. The child with vomiting alone could quite likely have some other condition. Many children present with gastro-intestinal symptoms when, in fact, the primary source of infection is not in the gastrointestinal tract and so a thorough clinical examination is mandatory. Breast feeding in the newborn period and during early infancy affords good protection against gastroenteritis and the factors accounting for this include:

Breast feeding

(1) Avoidance of serious bacterial contamination in preparing the feed.
(2) Lower stool pH with prevalence of lactobacilli which in some way help exclude gastrointestinal pathogens.
(3) Cells in the human milk which phagocytize pathogenic bacteria and viruses.
(4) Lactoferrin which inhibits the multiplication of coliforms.
(5) Secretory IgA which inhibits the invasion of pathogenic *E. coli* through the gastrointestinal mucosa. There are

33

also antibodies which provide some passive protection against virus infection.

Infecting agents causing childhood diarrhoea are shown in Table 3.1.

Table 3.1 Infective agents causing diarrhoea in children

Bacteria	Pathogenic *Escherichia coli*
	Shigella
	Salmonella
	Staph. aureus
	Campylobacter
Viruses	Rota virus
	Parvo virus-like agents
	Cytomegalovirus
Protozoa	*Giardia lamblia*
Helminths	*Ascaris lumbricoides* (roundworm)
	Trichuris (threadworm)
	Enterobius (pinworm)
	Toxocara
Mycosis	*Candida*

The most common pathogens in this country are usually the viruses which can be detected on electron microscopy followed by the well recognized bacterial pathogens. Threadworm and infestations seldom cause serious gastrointestinal upset.

Symptoms

Diarrhoea is the prevailing symptom. It should be remembered that babies will tend to have a bowel action after every feed and loose runny yellow stools from breast fed babies are quite normal. However, more than six stools per day would be considered abnormal, particularly if the stools are loose, green and slimy.

Fluid and electrolyte loss

The dangers of gastroenteritis are fluid and electrolyte loss which can occur very quickly in a small baby, especially if vomiting occurs in association with diarrhoea.

The severity of dehydration can be classified as follows:

(1) Mild – a reasonably well-looking baby. The anterior font- anelle may be slightly depressed. There is no significant loss in skin turgor. The baby may well be taking fluids in spite of the diarrhoea and there is a good urinary output.

(2) Moderate – An unwell baby showing lack of interest. Perfusion poor with cold extremities. Not tolerating fluids readily. Urine output poor. There are significant signs of dehydration with depressed fontanelle, loss of skin turgor, dryness of the mouth, lowered intra-ocular tension.

(3) Severe – A very ill child. Gross peripheral circulatory failure with peripheral cyanosis. Hyperventilation. Gross signs of dehydration. Oliguria or anuria.

Management The mild case of gastroenteritis can be treated at home but will require careful assessment of progress. Breast fed babies can be given clear fluids for a short period of time, up to 24 hours, and then breast feeding resumed. If solids are started it is best to omit these from the diet until the diarrhoea settles. It is important to enquire into the mother's diet as to whether she is ingesting foods that might precipitate loose stools in the baby such as fruits and curries or whether she is taking aperients.

Bottle fed babies, likewise, should be put on clear fluids and then regraded with first of all dilute formula feeds, regrading to full strength feeds over a period of 2–3 days according to tolerance.

Glucose electrolyte mixtures Glucose electrolyte mixtures are available and these are useful in outbreaks of severe diarrhoea. It is important to reconstitute them carefully. There is a great danger in telling patients how to make up their own glucose electrolyte mixture. One has experienced doctors who have told parents to make up mixtures which are far too hypertonic and, in turn, parents have got confused as to the portions of salt and water to add, ending up with a baby with hypernatraemia. In the absence of an available glucose electrolyte mixture it is quite reasonable to give boiled water sweetened with dextrose and for a short period of time babies with mild gastroenteritis will not run into severe electrolyte imbalance.

Antibiotics Antibiotics seldom have a place in the treatment of gastroenteritis, the mainstay of treatment being rehydration and maintenance of electrolyte balance. The natural history is that the pathogen will normally eliminate itself in the course of time and antibiotics either aggravate the diarrhoea or only serve to produce a resistant organism. There are a few instances where antibiotics are indicated, for example *Campylobacter* infections where erythromycin is indicated.

Hospital admission Those children retaining fluids with a good urinary output and no adverse clinical signs can be adequately treated at home but for the child with moderately severe dehydration who is in a state of negative fluid balance, hospital admission is required as intravenous fluid therapy may well be required. Most children's units will admit cases of gastroenteritis and it is probably better that they are admitted to such units rather than to fever hospitals since they have all the full facilities for care of the

35

child as a whole. This obviously would depend on the local facilities available.

Gastro-intestinal intolerances

Following gastroenteritis, problems can occur when milk is re-introduced. Lactose intolerance is one of the more common problems due to damage of the small bowel mucosa, leading to
Diagnosis impaired lactase production. It is a simple condition to diagnose by extracting a portion of the liquid fraction of the stool and testing it for reducing substances with a Clinitest tablet.
Treatment   Treatment of lactose intolerance is to exclude lactose from the diet so lactose-free milk is required. The duration of excluding lactose will vary according to the speed of recovery and usually it is advisable to avoid lactose for at least 6 months before attempting to re-introduce ordinary milk.

Other sugar intolerances do occur, including sucrose and fructose intolerance. These can be identified by sugar chromatography of the stools. Treatment is by exclusion of the relevant sugar from the diet.

Cow's milk protein intolerance

This has received much consideration in recent years. It may be associated with lactose intolerance complicating gastroenteritis. It varies in presentation and among the features are the following:

(1) Failure to thrive,
(2) Diarrhoea, often with blood in the stools,
(3) Vomiting, often just after a feed and associated with colicky abdominal pain,
(4) Skin rashes,
(5) Eosinophilia in the peripheral blood film.

At times it presents very abruptly after breast feeding has been stopped and cow's milk introduced. It seems more marked when raw cow's milk is introduced as opposed to formula feed. The
Diagnosis diagnosis should really be made by jejunal biopsy but where there is a strong clinical suspicion, it is reasonable to assume the diagnosis if there is a clinical response after excluding cow's milk from the diet. Among the preparations available for this condition are the following:

36

Prosobee,
Velactin,
Galactomin,
Wysobee,
Nutramigen and
Pregestimil.

It is strongly emphasized that these milks should only be prescribed for genuine cow's milk protein intolerance. The milks are very expensive and should not be used as a trial for minor feeding problems. Most children are usually able to tolerate cow's milk products by the age of 2 years.

MALABSORPTION

Coeliac disease

Sensitivity to gluten

Symptoms

Coeliac disease has a variable incidence, occurring in about 1 in 2000 children. Its cause is a sensitivity to gluten in wheat, rye, barley and oat germ, giving rise to villous atrophy in the small bowel. It is a condition that occurs in all ages but the most common time of presentation is between 9 months and 2 years of age. In many instances the presentation is classical with failure to thrive, offensive stools, anorexia and vomiting. The child is generally miserable, wasted and the abdomen is distended. The stools are bulky and offensive and it should be remembered that some children with coeliac disease may not have any change in bowel habit and, in fact, some may even be constipated. Unexplained iron deficiency anaemia may be another sign of coeliac disease in the otherwise well child. Developmental delay in a young infant can be one of the initial features before there is obvious failure to thrive. Children with short stature are often investigated for growth hormone deficiency but if they are below the 3rd centile in weight, it is more probable that they have malabsorption rather than any endocrine disorder.

Jejunal biopsy

Treatment

A definite diagnosis is a prerequisite before starting treatment and any child suspected of having coeliac disease should be referred for investigation including a jejunal biopsy.

Treatment is a gluten-free diet which should be adhered to rigidly throughout the child's growing years. Periodic lapses from the diet may not precipitate gross symptoms but may often contribute to the child reaching adult life with short stature. In the initial treatment of the disease it may be important to give a low fat diet and supplementing this with vitamins, in particular the fat-soluble ones. In some children there may be associated lactose intolerance due to the villous atrophy.

Coeliac
Society

Hospital dietitians are usually most helpful in advising parents on the diet. It may also be helpful for the family to join the Coeliac Society since this is often a source of useful advice.

Cystic fibrosis

Symptoms

This may cause profound failure to thrive due to lack of pancreatic enzymes. There may well be a history of recurrent respiratory tract infections. As opposed to coeliac disease where anorexia and vomiting are not uncommon, children with cystic fibrosis often eat exceedingly well but fail to gain weight. The stools are large, bulky and fatty. The diagnosis is confirmed

Sweat test

by performing a sweat test. Sweat sodium levels in excess of 60 mmol/l or sweat chlorides above 50 mmol/l are diagnostic of the condition.

Other malabsorption conditions

Giardia
lamblia

There are less common malabsorption conditions which include infestation with *Giardia lamblia*. Many patients may only have mild gastrointestinal upset with this but it can result in malabsorption. The condition responds well to metronidazole and when treating the patient it is important to treat the family as a whole since this may be a reservoir for further infestation.

Gastrointest-
inal allergies

Cow's milk protein intolerance can result in malabsorption as can other gastrointestinal allergies.

Blind loop
syndrome

Blind loop syndrome in the child following gastrointestinal surgery.

Traumatized
bowel

Traumatized bowel from previous non-accidental injury leading to malabsorption.

β-lipoprotein-
aemia

A-β-Lipoproteinaemia which is a rare inherited condition with an autosomal mode of inheritance. Malabsorption is due to the instability of the endoplasmic reticulum of the intestinal absorptive cells synthesizing the apoprotein of low density lipoprotein. In later childhood neurological manifestations develop including ataxia and retinitis pigmentosa.

Intestinal
lymphangi-
ectasia

Intestinal lymphangiectasia is a rare condition of the intestinal lymphatics. Other clinical signs of lymphactic obstruction may give a clue to the diagnosis in addition to gastrointestinal symptoms.

Toddler diarrhoea

This is a common source of concern. It occurs in children of 1–3 years. The child has often had gastroenteritis and, persists in having frequent loose stools but is otherwise quite healthy and gaining weight. Between 1 and 2 years children tend to put everything to their mouth and so the gastrointestinal tract is submitted to a variety of 'delicacies'. In the extreme, children with pica will even eat soil, leaves, worms or anything else they can find.

   Observation is the best course of action providing the child is healthy and there is no weight loss. It is very important to inform and reassure the parents of the nature of the condition. Should things be otherwise, further gastrointestinal investigation is necessary.

Chronic inflammatory bowel disease

Crohn's disease

Hitherto this was thought to be rare in children but in recent years gastroenterologists have been reporting an increased incidence. Crohn's disease (regional ileitis) can affect any part of the gut. The aetiology is unknown. It is very rare in children under the age of 6 years. Symptoms include failure to gain

Symptoms weight, poor growth, anorexia, abdominal distension, lethargy, fatigue and in the later stages abdominal pain and diarrhoea are the prevailing symptoms.

Diagnosis   The diagnosis is made by careful examination including proctosigmoidoscopy and biopsy. A barium enema should also be performed to demonstrate segmental lesions of ulceration, fissures and fistulas. A small bowel series should also be done.

Treatment   Treatment is mainly supportive with a high protein, low fat diet. A low oxalate intake is recommended in view of the high urinary oxalate level in patients with this disease. Corticosteroids and Salazopyrin are given for acute exacerbations.

Surgery   Surgery is indicated if there is intestinal obstruction or fistulae but resection of the lesions does not afford a cure. In the long term it should be remembered that patients with this disease

Malignant   have a forty times greater risk of developing malignant disease
disease   of the bowel.

Ulcerative colitis

Incidence This has an incidence of 2–6 cases per 100 000. It is more common in the second decade of life, although can occur at all ages. Approximately 10% of patients have relations with inflammatory bowel disease but there is not a definite mode of inheritance. Ulcerative colitis tends to be a more severe disease in children than adults.

Symptoms Symptoms include bloody diarrhoea with as many as 10–12 bowel actions a day associated with fever, abdominal cramps, anaemia, tachycardia, weight loss, oedema and hypoprotein-aemia. On examination the child looks apprehensive and ill. There is evidence of generalized malnutrition, often short stature, mouth ulceration and peripheral oedema. The abdomen may be mildly distended. Tenderness is often more marked in the left hypochondrium. Rectal examination is painful and may reveal blood and mucus on the glove. Microscopy of the stool will show blood and an excess of leukocytes.

Toxic megacolon Toxic megacolon is a serious complication of severe ulcerative colitis and is characterized by severe abdominal distension, tenderness and ileus. Associated features are arthritis, usually involving the large joints, cutaneous lesions including erythema nodosum and pyoderma gangrenosa. Iritis is a less common feature in children. Thrombophlebitis and hepa-titis tend to be rare complications as well.

Other complications

Diagnosis Diagnosis is confirmed by proctosigmoidoscopy showing spontaneous friability of mucosal bleeding and rectal biopsy is confirmatory. Barium enemas should be done in order to confirm proximal disease and to differentiate from Crohn's disease. It should not be performed during an acute exacer-bation of the disease as it may cause perforation.

Treatment Treatment – firstly it is important to discuss the nature of the disease with the parents and child. As regards specific medication, adrenocorticosteroids are useful in acute exacer-bations. They can either be given as ACTH gel by intermittent injection, prednisolone orally or by enema. It is thought that steroid enemas in children are not as effective as in adults.

Steroids

Salazopyrine Salazopyrine is used after remission has been induced as it reduces the likelihood of further exacerbation. The dosage is 50 mg/kg/day and it should be continued indefinitely. Gastric upsets can be avoided by using enteric coated tablets. Compli-cations of therapy include skin rashes, bone marrow suppres-sion and folic acid deficiency, but fortunately these are uncommon.

Surgery

Surgery – the main indications are profuse haemorrhage, toxic megacolon, perforation, obstruction, malignancy and chronic disablement with failure to grow. Growth retardation is an important consideration for surgery and it should be performed before the epiphyses are fused.

As chronic inflammatory bowel disease is uncommon it is usually wise to seek guidance from a paediatric or adult gastro-enterologist having a special interest in these disorders.

Congenital anomalies of the gastrointestinal tract

Congenital hypertrophic pyloric stenosis

Incidence

This occurs in approximately 1 in 150 male infants and 1 in 750 female infants. About 15% of cases have evidence of a familial incidence and there is a higher incidence among monozygotic twins.

Onset

Clinical manifestations seldom occur in the first week of life but usually in the second or third and occasionally as late as three months of life. At the onset the vomiting is not projectile but this evolves after a few days and is significant by one week. The vomiting most usually occurs during or just after a feed and the vomitus contains only the gastric contents except that these can occasionally be blood-stained. In spite of the vomiting the baby is eager to feed. The stools are usually small and infrequent and are often green due to starvation.

Projectile vomiting

Physical appearance

The physical appearance of the baby will depend on the severity of the condition. In the extreme the baby will be wasted and dehydrated. Visible peristalsis may be observed during a feed.

Diagnosis by palpation

Diagnosis is made by palpation of the pyloric tumour during feeding. The technique of this is important. Firstly the stomach should be emptied by passing a nasogastric tube. This will give some indication of gastric residue. During the test feed the baby should be examined from the left side with the 3rd and 4th fingers placed midway between the umbilicus and the lower edge of the liver, along the outer border of the rectus sheath. On deep palpation when the baby is relaxed a small, firm, olive-like mass can be felt and once this is definite the diagnosis is confirmed.

A barium meal is seldom needed to establish the diagnosis,

41

but it can be used when in doubt. Ultrasound may ultimately be the easiest confirmatory technique.

Treatment   Once the diagnosis is suspected, the child requires admission to hospital for confirmation of the diagnosis and replacement of fluid and electrolyte loss. It is important that
Surgery   surgery is not undertaken until full correction of the fluid balance of electrolytes has taken place. Pylorotomy (Rammstedt's operation) is the operation of choice. It carries a low mortality and the results are very satisfactory.

Mild   There are some babies, particular older ones, who have
obstruction   only mild pyloric obstruction in which case Eumydrin can be used but, it should not be used until the diagnosis is certain, as it may often mask symptoms which require further investigation.

Duodenal atresia

This is characterized by bile-stained vomiting in the newborn period. About 30% of patients with this condition have Down's syndrome. A plain X-ray of the abdomen shows a typical double bubble of the stomach and first part of the duodenum. Surgery is the treatment of choice.

Anomalies of rotation

These represent failure of the bowel to rotate in embryonic life and become fixed normally. Most often it is the caecum that fails to rotate into the right iliac fossa. The narrow mesenteric stalk which suspends the small intestine in the area of the superior mesenteric vessels is liable to volvulus giving rise to intestinal obstruction. The clinical picture is therefore one of acute intestinal obstruction in the first year of life.

Large bowel obstruction

Hirschsprung's disease

Cause   Hirschsprung's disease is the most common cause of obstruction of the colon. The disease results from absence of the ganglion cells in the bowel wall extending from the anus for a variable distance.
Clinical   Clinical symptoms vary from complete obstruction in the
symptoms   neonatal period to chronic constipation in the older child. In the

42

Newborn   newborn the symptoms may present from birth with failure to pass meconium or during the first week of life partial or incomplete intestinal obstruction with vomiting and abdominal distension. Rectal examination is followed by a characteristic gush of faeces and flatus, often giving temporary relief. Some neonates may, in fact, develop diarrhoea with toxic enterocolitis with profound dehydration and shock.

Older children   In the older child constipation and abdominal distension is the feature, with symptoms backdated to infancy. A large faecal mass is palpable per abdomen but on rectal examination the rectum is not dilated and is usually empty. The stools, when passed, are more like pellets. Seldom is there faecal soiling as compared to functional megacolon when this is very common.

Diagnosis   Diagnosis is made by rectal biopsy. Barium enema may also be helpful in ascertaining the extent of the disease.

Surgery   Treatment is surgical with resection of the aganglionic segment, usually with an initial colostomy or ileostomy followed by a re-anastomosis later to the anal canal.

Intussusception

This is a condition caused by one segment of the gut telescoping into the segment caudal to it, rather like turning a sock inside out. It is uncommon before 3 months and after 6 years of life. No specific cause has been determined but it is associated with adenovirus infection, gastroenteritis and occasionally Henoch–Schönlein's purpura. Anatomical lesions such as Meckel's diverticulum, a polyp or small bowel tumour act as an apex for intussusception. Most intussusceptions are ileocolic or ileoiliocolic.

Clinical signs   The clinical signs are sudden onset of severe paroxysmal abdominal pain in a previously well child. Between the paroxysms the child usually lies very still and looks pale and shocked. This appearance becomes more in evidence if the intussusception remains unreduced. Vomiting often occurs in the initial stages. The stools may be normal initially but after

'Redcurrant jelly' stools   some time may become blood-stained, giving the characteristic 'redcurrant jelly' stool.

Palpation   On palpation of the abdomen a mass may be palpable, often in the right hypochondrium. It is described as a sausage-shaped mass and may grow bigger during a paroxysm of pain.

Treatment   It is possible that some intussusceptions spontaneously reduce where others require reduction. This can be achieved by barium enema in some instances in liaison with a surgeon or by

43

Recurrence open surgery. Recurrence of an intussusception can occur and it is more likely to recur after reduction with an enema than by surgery.

Appendicitis

Rapid progress in children
This is the most common disease requiring surgery in childhood. It should be remembered that children progress to perforation far quicker than adults and because of this deaths which could be prevented regrettably still occur. The true incidence in childhood is not known. Males tend to predominate and the disease is uncommon under the age of 2 years and very rare under 1 year, most occurring in the adolescent age group range.

Cause
The cause is almost entirely due to obstruction of the lumen of the appendix by concretions or faecaliths. Ringworms are often found in the lumen but it is not thought that these cause the disease.

Symptoms
Appendicular obstruction produces mild colicky abdominal pain and reflex vomiting. As this is followed by inflammatory changes in the appendix, right lower abdominal pain develops which is accentuated by movement, including coughing and deep breathing.

Clinical signs
Fever, tachycardia and tenderness over the appendix at McBurney's point are cardinal signs. Unfortunately symptoms and signs are not always typical in children, some having persisting central abdominal pain and no pain in the right iliac fossa and vice versa. A retrocaecal or retro-ileal appendix may cause a child to produce an accentuated lumbar lordosis and tend to keep the right hip flexed owing to spasm of the psoas. A pelvic abscess may cause frequency of micturition owing to bladder irritation.

Particular care should be taken on examination of the abdomen as the anxious child will immediately splint the abdominal wall. Care should be taken in eliciting the site of maximal tenderness which, in the older child, is usually located over McBurney's point. Rebound tenderness can seldom be elicited before the age of 7–8 years, but pain produced on slightest movement is very suspicious of peritoneal irritation.

The signs are often difficult to elicit in children with abdominal pain and, if not acutely ill, it is reasonable to leave the child for an hour and then re-assess. However, the child under 5 years needs very careful assessment, since although appendicitis is rare, if perforation occurs it leads to widespread peritonitis.

Mesenteric lymphadenitis

This is a condition usually associated with upper respiratory tract infections. It often simulates acute appendicitis with fever, abdominal pain and vomiting. The pain is often spasmodic and usually peri-umbilical but can be anywhere, including the right iliac fossa. Tenderness is usually in the midline and may fluctuate from site to site. If there is any doubt the child should be admitted to hospital for further assessment since surgery is a lesser hazard than perforation of the undiagnosed appendix.

Differential diagnosis

Abdominal pain is a symptom in children of almost any disorder and so a full general physical examination is all the more important. Infections of the upper respiratory tract can be accompanied by abdominal pain and some of these have concurrent mesenteric adenitis. Right lower lobe pneumonia often occurs with predominant right-sided pain associated with muscular rigidity. Urinary tract infection can give abdominal pain and tenderness and gastroenteritis is often associated with crampy abdominal pain. Diabetic keto-acidosis in the undiagnosed diabetic child is not infrequently confused with an acute abdominal emergency presenting with acute abdominal pain and vomiting.

Urinalysis

Urinalysis is therefore mandatory in any patient with abdominal pain. Henoch Schönlein's purpura also gives rise to abdominal pain but often there are other features of the disease including skin manifestations and joint swelling. Abdominal pain may accompany rheumatic fever.

It should always be remembered that acute abdominal pain in children is often found with many of the common childhood diseases. It is important, therefore, to differentiate this from the acute surgical condition and whenever there is clinical doubt it

Hospital
admission

is quite reasonable to admit the child to hospital, at least for observation in case further investigation and other measures are required.

Urinary tract

Urinary tract infection – Congenital abnormalities of the renal tract – Glomerular disease – Renal tubular disorders

Urinary tract infection

Incidence of infection

Far too many children are diagnosed as having a urinary tract infection without objective proof, while others have a urinary tract infection which goes unrecognized. In about 2–20% of autopsies in children there is evidence of chronic pyelonephritis which has gone clinically unrecognized. In about 1–2% of female children (and about 6% of adults) who are apparently healthy without urinary tract symptoms, there is significant bacteriuria. However, it is fortunate that only a small proportion of these children go on to get chronic pyelonephritis and its recognized complications. Recent work (Ransley, et al.*) has shown that in some patients intrapapillary reflux occurs and is related to the development of chronic pyelonephritis. This probably accounts for some patients having recurrent urinary tract infections without the sequelae, while others proceed to show the radiological changes of chronic pyelonephritis with only a scant history of urinary tract infection.

Intrapapillary reflux

Diagnosis

Urinary tract infection is diagnosed entirely by examination of the urine. The findings are of significant bacteriuria with organisms cultured at greater than 10^5 orgs/ml with a pure growth of one organism. A growth of several organisms usually indicates contamination of the specimen on collection.

*Ransley, P. G. et al. (1977). Intrarenal reflux. Urol. Res., **5**, Part 1, 61

Additional findings may be proteinuria, haematuria and pus cells. Proteinuria and pus cells with negative bacterial culture can be found in febrile illnesses and dehydration (and in renal tuberculosis).

Collecting specimens

Obtaining a satisfactory specimen from children is not always straightforward. In infants a clean-catch specimen direct into a sterile container is ideal or, alternatively, apply a urine bag. Before applying a bag the genitalia should be cleansed with normal saline (and *not* any form of antiseptic as this will render the culture sterile). The older child may well oblige into a sterile receptacle. Having obtained the specimen it is important that it should be promptly despatched to the laboratory or stored in the fridge until collection. Agar-coated sticks (dip slides) can be used and the number of bacterial colonies cultured after an incubation period of 24 hours can be estimated against standard charts. These are particularly helpful in general practice where there may well be a problem of getting a specimen satisfactorily off to the laboratory.

Proof of infection is important since it colours the whole basis of future management. Genuine urinary tract infection not only requires appropriate treatment but in most instances investigation of the urinary tract is required and a complete follow-up must be made to see if the urine remains free from infection. It should be remembered that children may have symptoms suggestive of a urinary tract infection with dysuria and frequency but they are not always the result of bacterial infection and may be non-specific. When in doubt it is reasonable to send three consecutive specimens of urine to the laboratory, preferably taken early morning, and this will usually clarify the situation.

Clinical manifest- ations

Many children do not have overt symptoms. In the newborn there may be persistent neonatal jaundice or failure to thrive. Fever, irritability, vomiting and abdominal pain are not uncommon in a toddler and a relapse of enuresis in the older child is not uncommon. Urgency, frequency, dysuria and smelly urine occasionally with haematuria associated with high fever and loin pain are the symptoms seen in the older child as in the adult.

Management

Escherichia coli is the common pathogen causing urinary tract infection and most are sensitive to a sulphonamide or trimethoprim/sulphamethoxazole. Although most coliforms are sensitive to ampicillin, it is not ideally the first drug of choice since it encourages resistant organisms in the bowel which may re-infect the urinary tract with a resistent organism. A 2 week course of treatment is necessary followed 2 weeks later by a urine check to see that it has remained clear.

Radiological investigations

The indications for radiological investigation – intravenous pyelogram and micturating cystogram are as follows.

(1) A male child who has a urinary tract infection should be referred immediately for investigation since, apart from during the neonatal period, most infections in males are inevitably associated with some renal tract anomaly which may require surgical correction.

(2) More than one urinary tract infection in a girl should, likewise, be referred for investigation. Urinary tract infection does occur more frequently in girls and many have entirely normal urinary tracts but there are a significant number that do have abnormalities which require investigation and therefore a recurrence of infection is an important indication for further investigation.

Significance of micturating cystogram

Opinions differ as to whether all children require a micturating cystogram in addition to an intravenous pyelogram. Whilst in most instances if the intravenous pyelogram is normal with normal waters other abnormalities are probably unlikely. On the other hand it is possible in some instances to have a normal IVP yet a micturating cystogram will demonstrate abnormalities hitherto unshown. Such investigations are traumatic for the child and do involve a significant amount of radiation but are nevertheless important. Newer developments in ultrasound might hopefully limit the necessity for some of the X-ray investigations in the future.

Longterm chemotherapy

The child who has congenital renal abnormalities may well require to be on prophylactic therapy for 1–2 years. Often only a single daily dose is required in order to keep the urine clear. The child who has frequent recurrent urinary tract infections even though the IVP and micturating cystogram are normal, may likewise require a prolonged course of treatment. For the female child who has a normal urinary tract and only sporadic infections, it is quite reasonable to treat the infections as and when they arise.

Follow-up

Meticulous follow-up with regular urinary culture is very important. In the first instance accurate diagnosis of a urinary tract infection is vital in order to decide future management. Investigation of the urinary tract in order to elucidate any abnormality is important, as surgery may be required, for conditions such as for hydronephrosis or vesico-ureteric reflux

49

and some other abnormalities. Care in follow-up is vital since it is possible way of preventing hypertension and renal failure in adult life due to pyelonephritis.

Renal calculi

These are much less common in children than in adults and are twice as common in boys as in girls. The incidence is greater in the under-developed countries than in the Western world. Causes of nephrolithiasis include urinary tract infection which is associated with proteus infections as well as with urinary stasis due to congenital abnormalities, hypercalcaemia, cystinuria, hyperoxaluria and idiopathic causes. Most stones consist of calcium oxalate or phosphate or a mixture of both.

Management   Management consists of a high fluid intake, analgesia, treating urinary tract infection and investigation. Depending on the size of the calculus surgical removal may be required.

Congenital abnormalities of the renal tract

These are numerous and since many are rare only a selection are mentioned.

Renal agenesis

Unilateral renal agenesis occurs in about 1 in 2500 births. The single kidney is usually normal and the outlook therefore good. Bilateral renal agenesis constitutes the Potter syndrome occurring in about 1 in 3000 births. It is more common in males and is associated in pregnancy with oligohydramnios. There are extra-renal associations of abnormal facies with low-set ears and hypoplastic mandible, pulmonary hypoplasia often leading to pneumothorax and limb abnormalities.

Hydronephrosis

This is commonly due to pelvi-ureteric obstruction which is often a physiological obstruction due to abnormal muscular function of the ureter at that point. It may, on occasions, be due to an aberrant renal vessel.

Mega-ureter

This may or may not be associated with vesico-ureteric reflux or with ureteric obstruction. Occasionally a mega-ureter results from a ureterocele which is a congenital cystic ballooning of the distal portion of the ureter projecting into the bladder. Vesico-ureteric reflux may be primary or secondary. Primary reflux is due to a developmental anomaly with reflux resulting from the lack of valve-effect normally created by the passage of the ureter through the intravesical submucosal tunnel. Secondary reflux usually results from bladder outflow obstruction. The management of vesico-ureteric reflux has been controversial and depends on the degree of reflux. Since mild degrees of vesico-ureteric reflux are seldom associated with renal damage, surgery is not indicated but if associated with recurrent urinary tract infections it is important for the child to have longterm prophylactic chemotherapy as well as to advise frequent voiding and double micturition. Spontaneous regression of reflux occurs in over 50% of cases after the age of 5 years but this is unlikely if reflux is severe. For those cases surgery will be required to reimplant the ureters, a procedure which is usually accompanied by a high percentage of technical success. Because of these implications radiological investigation of urinary tract infection is important.

Vesico-ureteric reflux

Management

Regression

Surgery

Wilm's tumour

This usually occurs before the age of 5 with an average age of presentation of 3 years. It has associations with other congenital abnormalities including those of the genito-urinary tract and with hemi-hypertrophy. Some children have bilateral tumours, in which case the presentation is usually earlier in infancy. The tumour metastasizes to the lung and less commonly to the liver in addition to spreading along the regional lymph nodes.

Metastases

The clinical presentation is of an abdominal mass and there may be abdominal pain and sometimes vomiting and fever. The mass is smooth and firm and rarely crosses the midline.

The diagnosis is made radiologically. Treatment is nephrectomy even in the presence of pulmonary metastases as these may be sensitive to radiation and chemotherapy. The prognosis depends on the age and the stage of the tumour.

Nephrectomy

51

Glomerular disease

Acute post-streptococcal glomerulonephritis

β-Haemolytic streptococcus

This is the commonest form of nephritis and results from infection from a nephritogenic strain of group A β-haemolytic streptococcus. These infections are usually either in the upper respiratory tract or the skin. About 10–15% of those exposed to the infection from nephritic strains of streptococcus actually develop nephritis. There is evidence to suppose that prompt treatment of the initial infection significantly reduces the incidence of nephritis.

Clinical manifestations

These vary from the very mild, in patients who often never seek medical attention for diagnosis, to those that are severe. The majority present a fairly standard picture of a child who has had pharyngitis, scarlet fever or impetigo and then becomes unwell with puffy eyes, smokey-coloured urine, oliguria, abdominal pain, fever and malaise. Acute hypertension may occur giving rise to headache, vomiting and occasional fits. Congestive cardiac failure can occur and the child can develop acute pulmonary oedema.

Investigations

The urine is usually reddish-brown in colour (smokey). There is usually proteinuria, 30–100 mg/dl. Microscopy shows a varying number of red and white blood cells and a mixture of casts. The blood shows a mild normochromic anaemia due to haemodilution and there is a mild leukocytosis with a polymorph shift to the left. ESR is elevated.

The blood urea and the serum creatinine levels are increased and the serum sodium is often low due to haemodilution. In severe cases there may be disturbances in the acid–base equilibrium and hyperkalaemia.

Evidence of a β-haemolytic streptococcal infection can be shown by either a throat swab or elevation of the antistreptolysin O titres. The serum complement level is low for the first 10 days and returns to normal after 1 month.

Treatment
Mild cases

This depends on the severity of the disease. The child with a mild attack can be treated at home. Bed rest is not essential; if the child feels well he could be mobile. A 2 week course of penicillin is important to eradicate the β-haemolytic streptococcus and it is best if the diet has a low sodium and potassium content with ample carbohydrates and fats.

Hospital admission

The main cause of concern is the child who has significant malaise in association with heavy haematuria and who develops oliguria or hypertension. Under any of these cirumstances the child is best admitted to hospital. It should be remembered that these complications can occur suddenly and so careful surveillance is important.

Prognosis   The longterm prognosis for streptococcal glomerulonephritis is excellent provided that any complications are recognized early. Relapses can occur in the first 2 months of life especially if there is any intercurrent infection. Further attacks beyond this period are unusual unless there has been reinfection with another nephritogenic strain of organism.

Prevention   It is wise to swab all members of the family in close contact, taking nose and throat swabs, and if these grow β-haemolytic streptococci it is important to treat with a course of penicillin for 10 days.

Focal nephritis with recurrent haematuria (Berger disease)

This is a condition with recurrent haematuria which may be gross or microscopic, and is not associated with any recent infection of haemolytic streptococcus. The aetiology is unknown. The renal lesions often show mesangial deposits of immunoglobulins and complement. The condition should be investigated in order to exclude other renal pathology. No specific treatment is indicated. The prognosis is considered good.

Nephritis due to systemic lupus erythematosus

This is an uncommon disease in children but renal involvement should be considered in all cases of systemic lupus and is critical in considering the prognosis of the disease.

Nephritis of anaphylactoid purpura (Henoch–Schönlein)

Up to 50% of children with this condition develop glomerulonephritis and 2–3% will develop severe nephritis. It is therefore important to check the urine of all children with this disease for proteinuria and haematuria. When renal disease manifests after the other systemic symptoms have subsided or even develops late in the course of the disease, it usually heralds significant renal involvement. It is important, because of this phenomena, to regularly check the urine of these children until at least 6 months after the initial disease.

Glomerulonephritis associated with septicaemia

This may occur with bacterial endocarditis and generalized septicaemia arising from such conditions as acute osteitis and infected ventriculo-atrial shunts for hydrocephalus. The prognosis depends on the effective treatment of the underlying condition.

Haemolytic uraemic syndrome

Symptoms

This is an acute condition consisting of a micro-angiopathic haemolytic anaemia, thrombocytopenia and nephropathy. The condition follows gastroenteritis or a viral illness when the child develops pallor, purpura, irritability and oliguria. The urine may appear dark and yellow or smokey and there is moderate to severe proteinuria with microscopic haematuria and casts.

Hospital admission

Since these children are usually severely ill with risks of oliguria, hypertension and congestive cardiac failure, they require immediate admission to hospital. The prognosis is usually reasonably good with 95% of cases surviving the acute phase but the longterm prognosis is variable depending on the renal pathology.

Nephrotic syndrome

The most usual form of this disease in children is the minimal change lesion which is steroid-responsive but it should be remembered that other forms can occur in childhood which carry a less favourable prognosis.

Clinical features

The nephrotic syndrome is characterized by oedema, proteinuria and hypoproteinaemia associated with hyper-cholesterolaemia, hyperlipidaemia. The proteinuria is gross owing to the increased permeability of the glomerular basement membrane. The plasma proteins of low molecular weight such as albumin, IgG and transferrin, are excreted more readily than those of high molecular weight such as the lipoproteins. This relative clearance, inversely related to the molecular weight, is referred to as the selectivity of proteinuria.

Selectivity of proteinuria

Aetiology

The aetiology of nephrotic syndrome is unknown but the HLA histocompatibility antigen B-12 is common in children with minimal change lesion as is a history of atopy. The common age of incidence is 2–7 years. Over 80% of children have the minimal change lesion as opposed to less than 20% of adults.

The onset of oedema occurs with an increase of 10–20% in bodyweight associated with low urine output. A preceding

Clinical manifest- ations	minor upper respiratory tract infection is not uncommon. The child is usually not acutely ill. In addition to puffiness of the eyes and face there is often ascites and pleural effusions. The blood
Susceptibility to infection	pressure is usually normal. There is a significant *susceptibility to infection* particularly due to *Streptococcus pneumoniae* as well as organisms including *Haemophilus influenzae* and coliforms. Venous and arterial thrombosis may be a serious complication as well as shock induced by sudden diuresis.
Treatment	There are just a few cases who remit spontaneously but most require active treatment. The main drug of choice is
Prednisolone	prednisolone (2 mg/kg/24 h up to 60 mg a day). The response is usually within the first 2 weeks of starting therapy and if there is no response after 1 month of treatment, this drug is likely to be ineffective. In most cases proteinuria ceases after 1 month or sooner and after this the steroid dosage can be progressively reduced and after a 2 week period of being totally protein-free, it can be stopped entirely.

In view of the likelihood of infection, it is important that while the child has proteinuria and is on high doses of steroids, he should be prescribed a prophylactic dose of penicillin.

While most cases of nephrotic syndrome respond to corticosteroids, many relapse and require further courses of steroids and some require longterm steroid therapy over a period of 1–2 years in order to keep them in remission. It is important where possible to give the dose on alternate days in order to avoid

Other drugs undue suppression of growth hormone. Other drugs that have been used in treatment of this condition, include cyclophosphamide, azathioprine and chlorambucil but these are only usually prescribed by either a paediatrician or a paediatric nephrologist.

Prognosis Most have a good prognosis, i.e. those with minimal change lesions. Renal biopsy is usually thought not necessary providing there is a good response to prednisolone. If, however, the response to steroids is poor, renal biopsy might well be necessary in order to elucidate the histology and the prognosis will depend on this finding.

Renal tubular disorders

Renal glycosuria

A hereditary defect in glucose transport giving rise to variable glycosuria in the presence of a *normal* blood glucose level.

55

Disorders in which other sugars or reducing substances appear in the urine should be excluded and these include fructosuria, galactosuria, sucrosuria, maltosuria and pentosuria.

Renal tubular acidosis (RTA)

This consists of a metabolic acidosis, hyperchloraemia, in a patient with a normal glomerular filtration rate. The cause is an impaired ability of the kidney to maintain a normal plasma bicarbonate due to defective acidification of the urine or impaired reabsorption of bicarbonate. The urine has a pH inappropriately high in relation to the metabolic acidosis.

Defective acidification of urine

Two forms

There are two main physiologically distinct forms of renal tubular acidosis, although intermediate forms exist. These are (1) distal renal tubular acidosis (type I) and (2) proximal renal tubular acidosis (type II). Both occur as primary abnormalities in urinary acidification. They can occur as a secondary disorder to systemic disease and intoxication.

Primary distal renal tubular acidosis in early childhood may be inherited as an autosomal recessive condition or occur in later childhood as an autosomal dominant condition. In other cases the disease may occur sporadically. Proximal renal tubular acidosis is more commonly related to systemic disorders

Clinical features

The clinical features are related to the electrolyte disturbances. The symptoms include vomiting, failure to thrive and polyuria.

Treatment

Treatment is by giving alkali plus potassium either by giving sodium bicarbonate with potassium supplements or giving Scholl's mixture (citric acid plus sodium citrate). Longterm follow-up is obviously essential.

Fanconi's syndrome

This consists of osteomalacia with refractory rickets growth retardation, the proximal type of renal tubular acidosis, renal glycosuria, hyperphosphatasia and hypophosphataemia, generalized amino aciduria, proteinuria, ketonuria plus excessive excretion of sodium and potassium ions, uric acid and calcium. It is a familial disease but may result from poisoning and can be associated with other metabolic disorders.

Clinical manifest- ations

The clinical manifestations are of an infant developing symptoms at the age of 6 months of growth retardation, oedema and dehydration.

Treatment   Treatment consists of treating the electrolyte disturbances and vitamin D.

Nephritogenic diabetes insipidus

This is a congenital hereditary disorder in which the kidneys do not respond to antidiuretic hormone, giving rise to polydipsia and polyuria. It is a disease mainly of males and has an X-linked recessive mode of inheritance. The unresponsiveness of the distal tubule and collecting duct to vasopressin is probably the primary defect.

Clinical manifest-ations   Polydipsia and polyuria from birth are the clinical manifestations, together with poor growth, dehydration and constipation. Permitting an adequate fluid intake is important. Hydrochlorothiazide with a low sodium intake helps reduce the polyuria but the exact mode of action is unknown.

5 Fits in childhood

Neonatal fits – Febrile fits – Epilepsy – Infantile spasms – Differential diagnosis of peculiar turns

Neonatal fits

These are usually multifocal and at times can be difficult to differentiate from normal baby movements, especially if the baby is irritable. Careful observation usually discriminates the two as well as does the background history. An apnoeic attack can sometimes be the sole manifestaiton of a fit. The common causes of neonatal fits are:

Causes

(1) Severe anoxia
(2) Cerebral haemorrhage
(3) Trauma
(4) Biochemical causes which include hypoglycaemia, hypocalcaemia and hypomagnesemia
(5) Infection – meningitis, septicaemia.

Treatment

Treatment depends on the cause. The cerebrally irritable baby following a traumatic delivery can be sedated with chloral hydrate or phenobarbitone and actual convulsions treated by

(1) Phenobarbitone 3 mg/kg bodyweight
(2) Paraldehyde 0.1 ml/kg bodyweight
(3) Diazepam 0.25 mg/kg bodyweight

Hypoglycaemia can largely be prevented by early feeding and if it still occurs can be corrected by either oral or intra-

59

venous glucose. Hypocalcaemia can be corrected by oral or intravenous calcium gluconate though the latter must be administered with care and hypomagnesemia can be treated with intramuscular magnesium sulphate. The control of neonatal fits is important. The prognosis depends on the underlying pathology.

Febrile fits

Incidence

These occur in 3–5% of all children mostly between the ages of 6 months and 5 years, peaking at 2–3 years and occasionally persisting to 6–8 years of age. Boys are more susceptible than girls and there is an increased susceptibility in some families. In

Rise in body temperature

nearly all cases the fit has occurred after a sudden rise in body temperature as a result of infection. It is important to obtain a good history of events leading up to the fit and to perform a thorough physical examination to elicit the source of infection. It

Meningitis

should be remembered always that some children who present with febrile fits might have meningitis. While, in most instances

Risk of underlying condition

the fit occurs as a complication of an otherwise benign febrile illness, all other diagnostic possibilities should be considered. These include intracranial injury, haemorrhage, encephalopathy, poisoning, hypoglycaemia, tetany, hypertensive encephalopathy and anoxia.

Hospital admission

Most children with their first febrile fit tend to be admitted to hospital, many because the parents have brought them directly to the Accident and Emergency Department without consulting their general practitioner. The majority are admitted directly because of the anxiety it engenders in the parents and children under the age of 1 year usually undergo lumbar puncture since signs of meningitis at that age can be difficult to elicit. As far as other children are concerned, lumbar puncture is only performed when there are genuine clinical indications.

Re-admission for subsequent fits is not mandatory provided there are no signs of meningitis or any other serious underlying illness and the child can well be looked after at home.

Careful explanation to the parents of the nature of febrile fits is essential. Although a seizure, relatively few children go on

Prevention

into adult life with fits. They are purely associated with fever and therefore keeping the child cool when febrile with tepid sponging and antipyretics is the important preventative measure.

Fits in childhood

Management   During the fit it is important to turn the child on his side to maintain the airway and usually this is all that is required. Most

Prolonged fit febrile fits only last a few minutes but a prolonged febrile fit is a matter of concern, since status is a situation where the child can incur damage and so it is a matter of urgency to stop the fit, by cooling the child and administering paraldehyde or diazepam.

Anti-convulsants   Prophylaxis with anticonvulsants is controversial. It is reasonable to give these to children who have had either very severe or very frequent fits. Phenobarbitone has been the drug of choice in the past, but some children do react adversely to this, becoming hyperactive and aggressive. Sodium valproate has been given more recently and although it has no substantial advantage in preventing the seizures, it may well have fewer disadvantageous side-effects.

Prognosis   Overall the outlook for febrile seizures is good but there are a small percentage of children who do develop subsequent epilepsy later and there is some correlation with temporal lobe epilepsy in a child who has had prolonged febrile seizures.

Epilepsy

Causes In the majority of cases there is no established cause but among the recognized causes are the following:

(1) Cerebral damage from anoxia or trauma,
(2) Congenital cerebral malformations,
(3) Genetically determined disorders,
(4) Biochemical causes.

     It is important to endeavour to establish a cause because the condition itself might be amenable to treatment as is true of phenylketonuria, or it might be a condition where there are genetic implications, in which case genetic counselling for future family planning is very important.

Grand mal seizures

Symptoms These are the classical generalized convulsions. In children fewer than one third describe an aura. Vague prodromal symptoms such as irritability, mental dullness, headache, gastrointestinal symptoms, may forwarn parents of an impending fit. The onset of the fit is abrupt with the tonic phase coinciding with loss of consciousness. Micturition and less frequent, defaecation may follow as a result of contraction of the

61

abdominal muscles. The tonic phase usually lasts about 30 seconds and is followed by the clonic phase which is of variable duration. In the post-ictal state the child usually goes off into a deep sleep and on waking often complains of headache and there may be confusion and occasionally automatism or transient paresis. Nocturnal epilepsy can occur without the patient being aware of it. Blood on the pillow, a bitten tongue, headache in the morning, unexplained bed-wetting are symptoms which can be relevant.

Nocturnal epilepsy

An explanation of epilepsy to the parents and the child is most important. Many children who have epilepsy go into adult life and have no further fits and so there are reasonable grounds for cautious optimism. Swimming can be allowed but the presence of a competent life-saver is important. Climbing high ladders is best avoided as is riding a bicycle on a main road without and escort. Otherwise one would encourage such children to lead as normal a life as possible.

Restrictions

Medication

The pros and cons of medication should be carefully weighed up before embarking on anticonvulsants. If a child has had a solitary fit it is better to wait and see whether the fits are likely to be recurrent before immediately embarking on therapy. The choice of medication for grand mal seizures includes a wide range of drugs which include the following:

(1) Sodium valproate — this is being used more extensively in childhood epilepsy since it affords good control with minimal side-effects. There have, however, been reports of liver damage particularly in children on multiple therapy containing other anticonvulsants.

(2) Phenytoin — previously an extensively used drug. It is important that the therapeutic dose is correct for the child's age and weight and it is important to monitor blood levels since excessively high levels produce toxicity with nystagmus and slurred speech and low levels poor control. There are other side-effects including gingival hypertrophy and hirsutism which can be troublesome.

Fits in childhood

(3) Carbamazepine   can be used if phenytoin is not tolerated and is effective for focal and temporal lobe seizures.

(4) Mysoline   can be used alone or in combination with phenytoin. It can cause gastric upset on initial dosage and irritability and drowsiness.

(5) Phenobarbitone   although used extensively for many years, it is used far less at present, particularly in young children where it is often tolerated badly, causing hyperactivity and aggression often accompanied by poor learning. It tends, at present, to be used more for neonatal convulsions and febrile fits. It has little place in grand mal epilepsy.

Prognosis   Idiopathic epilepsy in childhood tends, on the whole, to have quite a good prognosis. Recurrence of fits can occur during puberty and for this reason it is sometimes reasonable to continue anticonvulsant therapy until the child has reached adulthood.

Petit mal

Symptoms   This manifests itself as blank spells due to transient loss of consciousness lasting for a few seconds, often associated with an upward rolling of the eyes and occasionally with quivering of the trunk. Girls are more commonly affected than boys. It rarely occurs before the age of 3 and usually disappears by puberty. There is seldom any intellectual impairment but a sustained series of attacks can produce a lapse in concentration. Attacks can be provoked by hyperventilation or exposure to a blinking light. This can be useful in provoking an attack in the clinic in a child presenting with a suspicious history.

Treatment   Ethosuximide has always been the drug of choice for most cases of straightforward petit mal. It can produce drowsiness, skin rashes, hiccup and occasionally blood dyscrasis. For this reason some recommend periodic blood counts that check there are no adverse affects.

Sodium valproate is now more commonly used in petit mal. It is particularly useful if petit mal occurs in conjunction with grand mal seizures.

63

Prognosis Petit mal which is uncomplicated has an excellent prognosis. There are some children who have both petit and grand mal seizures, the latter often manifesting after the petit mal has been controlled. The outlook for these cases is less favourable, often presenting difficulties of control and mental impairment.

Psychomotor attacks of temporal lobe epilepsy

Symptoms These are curious fits and often difficult to recognize. They present as purposeful but inappropriate movements or acts which are complicated and repetitive. There may be a brief aura with the child crying and signalling for help. The clinic picture of an attack varies widely and may include a period of staring and absence rather like petit mal but usually more prolonged. The patient is usually active during an attack. The activity may consist of movements of one part of the body such as stretching out of an arm or turning the head and eyes to one side, grimacing, biting and smacking the lips and swallowing movements. Peculiar behaviour and sudden spells of uncontrolled laughter may occur. In spite of this the patient is seldom completely out of touch and can answer questions, usually does not fall to the ground and has some recollection of his experience. The patient may have hallucinations or hear and smell something that does not exist. Some of these can be recalled by the child but often not, and they may produce alarm particularly if they occur at night when they may be associated with sleep walking. Other symptoms may include vertigo, nausea, headache and abdominal pain. It should be remembered that many

History of children with psychomotor epilepsy had a previous history of
febrile fits severe or frequent febrile fits.

The e.e.g. may be normal and changes may only be found if sleep is induced during the tracing.

Treatment Treatment.

(1) Carbamazepine – this may initially produce fatigue, dizziness, ataxia and diplopia but these effects can be avoided by starting with a small dose. Often grand mal seizures occur with psychomotor epilepsy and other anticonvulsants are sometimes needed to control these such as phenytoin, mysoline or sodium valproate.

(2) Sulthiame – this can also be used but it is thought to be less effective than carbamazepine but is worth trying if carbamazepine is ineffective. A troublesome side-effect of sulthiame is hyperventilation.

64

(3) Neurosurgery has been shown to be effective in certain selected cases of temporal lobe and intractable epilepsy.

Myoclonic and akinetic seizures

These may occur in conjunction with other forms of epilepsy or they may occur alone. The akinetic seizure is associated with sudden generalized loss of postural tone while myoclonic jerks are usually associated with a single group of muscles, are unilateral and may include loss of consciousness. The e.e.g. often shows a spike wave pattern similar to that of petit mal.

These seizures are frequently associated with degenerative disorders of the central nervous system and are difficult to control.

Treatment (1) Nitrazepam is effective but it should be remembered that it can precipitate grand mal seizures and so should be combined with suitable therapy for such. It can also induce increased salivation and bronchial secretion.

(2) Sodium valproate

(3) Clonazepam – this may produce drowsiness, fatigue, dizziness, muscular hypotonia and hypersalivation in infants as well as paradoxical aggression and irritability.

Infantile spasms

'Lightening attacks'

Clinical features

These are otherwise known as 'lightening attacks' or Salaam attacks. They occur mainly in the first year of life and the common clinical features are of mass myoclonus with dropping of the head and flexion of the arms. The attacks are repetitive and up to several hundred times a day. Children with this disorder can be divided roughly into two groups:

(1) Those with subnormal development or with seizures occuring before the age of 4 months are likely to have either major congenital cerebral defect or some other serious organic cause. The outlook for these children is poor and one of developmental retardation.

(2) Those in whom the seizures occur after 6 months, during which time there has been normal development, in which an encephalitis or an underlying defect in cerebral metabolism is the likely cause.

The outlook for infantile spasms overall is poor with only

about 10% of the second group having normal intellectual ability. In those with a chance of normal development there is urgency in establishing a diagnosis and starting treatment because undue delay significantly lessens the prognosis. The E.e.g. suspicion of infantile spasms is one of the few indications for an urgent e.e.g. The pattern of the tracing in this condition is typical giving a so-called hypsarrhythmic pattern.

Treatment   ACTH given in high doses over a period of 2 weeks, or if necessary up to 1 month until the seizures cease, is the standard treatment. Prednisolone can be given but ACTH is still thought to be preferable. Most cases will have some improvement and in those that respond well the fits will cease and the e.e.g. will return to a less abnormal pattern.

Differential diagnosis of peculiar turns

In most instances a case history will give a fair indication of the type of fit the child is getting or, indeed, whether the child is having a fit at all. There are, however, other conditions that should be considered.

(1) Cardiovascular

Vasovagal attacks
    (a) Vasovagal attacks or syncope – is usually seen in susceptible individuals. The patient is pale and sweating, is found to have a bradycardia and recovers when sat on the ground with the head down. Occasionally there are some who have a profound vasovagal attack giving rise to cerebral anoxia and a subsequent fit.

Cardiac arrhythmias
    (b) Cardiac arrhythmias – may give rise to a low cardiac output and can give rise to cerebral anoxia and hence a fit.

Breath-holding
(2) Breath-holding attacks are seen in young children from about 9 months to 4 years. These attacks are usually precipitated by an unpleasant experience or if the child is being thwarted and therein cries with a sound against a closed glottis, holding his breath until he becomes cyanosed and some may lose consciousness. Some of these children may have a resulting anoxic fit. Occasionally these episodes are difficult to differentiate from epilepsy. An e.e.g. in these circumstances can be helpful.

Poisons and
drugs

(3) Intoxications of poisons and drugs may produce fits. Anti-histamines and chlorpromazine lower the threshold of convulsions.

Tantrums and
imaginary fits

(4) Non fits: there are circumstances where parents vividly describe fits in their children but in fact no medical person has ever witnessed them. These can be tantrums or behaviour spasms which are interpreted as fits or sometimes there is a perverse parent who will prefabricate the whole story. These situations can be very difficult to elicit the true facts and in the long-run patient observation usually clarifies the situation.

Heart disease in children

Innocent murmurs – Basic cardiac parameters – Congestive cardiac failure – Ventricular septal defect – Patent ductus arteriosus – Atrial septal defect – Co-arctation of the aorta – Transposition of the great vessels – Tetralogy of Fallot – Pulmonary stenosis – Aortic stenosis – Truncus arteriosus – Tricuspid atresia – Precautions against infection

Although cardiac conditions in children are relatively uncommon, they do engender much concern, and the paediatrician's time is spent in seeing either those with genuine cardiac conditions or those who have been referred as they have been discovered to have a heart murmur. Paediatric cardiology is very much a specialist entity and so most children with recognized cardiac disease are usually under the care of a paediatric cardiologist. It is proposed to deal only with the more common conditions that are encountered.

Innocent or functional murmurs

These are murmurs associated with no demonstrable abnormality of the cardio-vascular system and are found in at least 30% of normal children. The characteristics are of a healthy child with no cardiac symptomatology who is found incidentally to have a murmur. The features of such murmurs are listed below.

Characteristic features

(1) Relatively low intensity.
(2) The murmur is localized to a small area of the precordium and does not radiate.

69

(3) The murmur is of short duration.

(4) It is vibratory or 'musical' in quality in some instances.

A murmur that is present on exercise but disappears on resting and one which disappears on deep inspiration is probably functional. Some murmurs are due to a venous hum which is a systolic murmur flowing into diastole, heard mainly over the aortic area. The murmur is soft and unlike that of a patent ductus arteriosus and never accentuates in diastole. Pressure on the jugular vein on turning the head reduces the intensity of the murmur.

Still's   Still's murmur is an innocent murmur heard between the ages of 3 and 7 years. It is a musical systolic ejection murmur of brief duration and heard down the left lower sternal edge. It is often accentuated in fever, exercise and excitement.

Supra-clavicular murmurs   Supraclavicular murmurs are probably due to turbulence from the brachiocephalic vessels. They are often heard maximally above the right clavicle and in the suprasternal notch when the patient is sitting erect. They disappear on hyper-extension of the shoulders.

Cardio-respiratory murmurs   Cardiorespiratory murmurs are probably produced by the impact of the heart against the lungs. The murmur is superficial, high pitched and well localized. The murmur is often intermittent and fluctuates with respiration.

Since the success of treating cardiac conditions has consistently improved over the years, it is important that children with heart murmurs are carefully assessed. The majority leave little reason on clinical grounds to suspect that they are other than innocent in nature but those in which some doubt exists should be referred for a paediatrician's opinion and he in turn can seek a paediatric cardiologist's opinion if required. The chest X-ray and e.c.g. are valuable in assessing the child since obviously in innocent murmurs these are quite normal. The e.c.g. of a child has to be interpreted according to the age and tables are available for interpreting the complex signs relative to age in most paediatric cardiology textbooks.

CONGENITAL HEART DISEASE

Aetiology   The prevalence is in the order of 8 per thousand live births with a range from 0.5–21 per thousand. The aetiology in most instances is not clear but there are recognized associations such as rubella, certain hereditary disorders and syndromes, some drugs and irradiation.

Basic parameters

Pulse   In infancy and childhood the pulse, blood pressure and respiratory rate will vary according to age. The resting pulse of the newborn is in the order of 125/min with a range of 70–190/min, at 2 years 110/min with a range of 80–130/min, and at 10 years

Blood pressure   90/min with a range of 70–110/min. Blood pressures in infancy are of the order of 80/50 in the newborn, 95/60 at the age of 2 years and 105/70 at the age of 10 years. It is important that the appropriately sized cuff should be used, covering two-thirds of

Respiration rates   the upper arm. Resting respiration rates are 30–40/min in the newborn, 25–30/min at the age of 2 and 20–25/min at the age of 10.

Chest X-ray   The chest X-ray of the newborn will show a cardiac shadow occupying up to 50% of the transverse diameter. The superior mediastinum may be widened owing to a thymic shadow. The e.c.g. of the newborn shows right axis and right ventricular dominance and during childhood there is progressive change from right ventricular dominance to LV dominance of the adult pattern.

Table 6.1 Relative frequency of congenital heart lesions in two age groups*

Lesion	Percentage of total lesions	
	Infants	*Others*
Ventricular septal defect	28.3	15.0
Patent ductus arteriosus	12.5	15.5
Atrial septal defect	9.7	16.0
Coarctation of the aorta	8.8	8.0
Transposition of the great vessels	8.0	2.0
Tetralogy of Fallot	7.0	15.5
Pulmonary stenosis	6.0	15.0
Aortic stenosis	3.5	5.0
Truncus arteriosus	2.7	–
Tricuspid atresia	1	1.0
Others	12.5	7.0

*(Hamish Watson, Paediatric Cardiology, 1968)

The diagnostic and surgical techniques for congenital heart disease have greatly advanced in recent years. It should be remembered that most children with congenital heart disease can be successfully treated and the longterm prognosis after surgery is encouraging although some conditions still

Importance
of early
reference

await longterm appraisal. In the newborn it is most important, once lesion is suspected, to seek a paediatric cardiological opinion immediately. This is because the risks of cardiac catheterization and surgery are much less when the baby is still in reasonable condition than when serious difficulties have arisen.

Congestive cardiac failure

Symptoms and
signs

The symptoms and signs of congestive cardiac failure in infants are dyspnoea with intercostal recession; difficult feeding, sweating and poor colour. In chronic congestive failure there may be deformity of the chest with widening of the AP diameter, and due to cardiomegaly there may be a precordial bulge. Other features are failure to thrive or inappropriate weight gain due to fluid retention, cyanosis, tachycardia, gallop rhythm and hepatomegaly.

CLINICAL ASPECTS OF THE MORE COMMON CONGENITAL HEART LESIONS

Ventricular septal defect (VSD)

The larger defects present in the neonatal period whereas the small defects are usually diagnosed on routine medical examination later in infancy or childhood. It is not uncommon for there to be no abnormal signs at birth as, although the VSD is present, the high foetal pulmonary vascular resistance prevents significant left-to-right shunting. During the first few weeks of life as the pulmonary vascular resistance falls, so the left-to-right shunt increases, a murmur appears and the baby may develop congestive heart failure.

Left-to-right
shunt

Clinical signs

In the uncomplicated situation the shunt is left-to-right and the child is pink. The first and second heart sounds are normal. There is usually a pansystolic murmur audible down the left sternal edge often accompanied by a precordial thrill. If the shunt is considerable the murmur is often transmitted to the back and at the apex there is a mid-diastolic murmur due to the increased flow across the mitral valve.

The chest X-ray shows mild to moderate cardiomegaly with increased pulmonary plethora. The e.c.g. usually shows biventricular hypertrophy with prominent Q and R waves in the left precordial leads which show left ventricular dominance.

Spontaneous
closure

The natural history of ventricular septal defects is that 50–60% of them close spontaneously in the first year of life.

Even in an infant with congestive cardiac failure, provided that this has been well controlled medically, it may close spontaneously. For the remainder, if any significant shunt persists, surgical closure will have to be considered.

Surgery
For the infant with intractible cardiac failure not controlled by digoxin and diuretics, surgery may have to be undertaken as an emergency procedure. In the past, banding of the pulmonary artery was done to reduce the pulmonary blood flow but at present the trend is for primary closure of the defect.

Pulmonary hypertension
While a high percentage of VSDs will close spontaneously, those that remain with a significant left-to-right shunt, risk developing pulmonary hypertension. The disappearance of the murmur may not always indicate that the defect has closed but rather that the shunt has ceased because of balancing of the pressures on both sides of the heart, eventually

Reverse shunt
leading to a reverse shunt from right-to-left, and irreversible pulmonary hypertension known as the Eisenmenger syndrome. Hence there is a need to assess such children carefully. The

Clinical signs of pulmonary hypertension
essential clinical signs of pulmonary hypertension include the onset of cyanosis, lack of growth, fatiguability. The lessening or disappearance of the systolic murmur and accentuation of the pulmonary second sound may be accompanied by a pulmonary systolic ejection click. There may be a palpable right ventricular impulse and the chest X-ray shows cardiomegaly and the lung fields have lost their plethora and show the 'tree in winter' appearance of pulmonary hypertension. The e.c.g. shows either biventricular or right ventricular hypertrophy.

Patent ductus arteriosus

Spontaneous closure
During the first 48 hours of life it is not uncommon to hear a systolic murmur in a neonate due to persistent patent ductus arteriosus. The majority of these close spontaneously but there are occasionally premature babies with respiratory distress syndrome who have a large patent ductus that requires closure during the neonatal period. It should be remembered in neonates that severe congestive cardiac failure may not be due to a complex cardiac lesion, but where due to a large patent ductus early diagnosis and ligation will lead to a good outcome.

Drugs
Drugs have been found to have an affect on the patency of the ductus arteriosus. Rising arterial PO_2 levels normally lead to closure of the ductus. Indomethacin has been found to produce closure of the ductus while prostaglandin E will keep the duct open and this can be useful therapeutically if the baby has a

lesion in which life depends on the patency of the duct.

Clinical signs Clinical signs are of a late systolic murmur flowing into a diastole usually maximally heard in the left infraclavicular region. There may be a palpable thrill in the second left inter-costal space. The pulse is characteristically jerky due to a wide pulse pressure and a Corrigan pulsation can be seen at times in the neck.

The chest X-ray may show a normally or moderately sized heart depending on the degree of shunt, a prominent pulmonary conus and increased pulmonary plethora. The e.c.g. is most likely to be normal in uncomplicated cases or to show left ventricular hypertrophy.

Treatment In the neonate indomethacin has been shown to hasten the closure of the duct. In older children surgical ligation is usually required.

Since many children who are discovered to have a patent ductus arteriosus are entirely asymptomatic, the parents may question the wisdom of surgical closure. Overall there is a 23 year reduction in life expectancy in males and a 28 year reduction in females if the lesion is left unclosed. Very few will close spontaneously after infancy and surgery for this condition carries a low mortality and morbidity.

Atrial septal defect

This defect can be separated into four types:

(1) Patent foramen ovale,
(2) Ostium secundum defect,
(3) Ostium primum defect,
(4) Ostium primum defect with a common atrioventricular canal.

Patent foramen ovale

80% close spontaneously after birth and isolated patency is of no haemodynamic significance unless associated with other abnormalities.

Ostium secundum defect

This is a defect which is seldom associated with defects of the AV valves. Depending on size there is a large shunt of blood from

Atrial shunt left to right at atrial level giving rise to a considerable increase in pulmonary blood flow. Since the pulmonary vascular resistance is higher in the neonatal period and the right ventricle relatively thick, there are seldom signs of this lesion in early infancy. Most children with atrial septal defects are discovered on routine examination, the child having been asymptomatic. Occasionally some children will have a history of recurrent pneumonitis.

Clinical signs
    The pulse is normal or of low amplitude. The jugular venous pressure is not raised unless there is associated tricuspid incompetence or congestive cardiac failure. The heart is clinically normal in size in most instances or slightly enlarged and there may be a palpable right ventricular impulse. There is a systolic ejection murmur maximal in the pulmonary area due to increased pulmonary blood flow. The first heart sound is normal but usually the second heart sound is widely split. This persists throughout both phases of respiration. Occasionally there is a mid-diastolic murmur due to torrential flow across the tricuspid valve.

    Chest X-ray shows a normal, or slightly enlarged heart with an increased right atrial and right ventricular shadow. The pulmonary artery is large, while the aorta and left ventricle are relatively small. The lung fields show pulmonary plethora.

Adult complications
    The e.c.g. shows right axis deviation and partial right bundle branch block. The majority of children are asymptomatic but in adult life there is the risk of pulmonary hypertension, cardiac arrhythmias, tricuspid incompetence, congestive cardiac failure and infective endocarditis. For this reason

Surgical closure
surgical closure is recommended in most instances and this is usually a straightforward procedure with a low mortality and morbidity. Rarely arrhythmias may develop later in life even after surgical correction.

Ostium primum defect

This is a lesion situated in the lower part of the atrial septum and extends to involve the endocardial cushions, particularly the mitral valve, where there is usually a cleft in the anterior leaflet.

Clinical signs
    There are many children who are asymptomatic and the condition is only detected on routine medical examination. Occasionally some children have a history of fatigue or recurrent pneumonitis. On examination the signs may be identical to that of an ostium secundum defect with a pulmonary

systolic ejection murmur and fixed splitting of the second heart sound. If, however, there is significant mitral incompetence, then there is an additional pansystolic murmur maximal at the apex and radiating round the axilla.

The chest X-ray shows a normal or enlarged heart with biventricular enlargement. The pulmonary conus is enlarged and there is pulmonary plethora.

The e.c.g. shows *left* axis deviation with biventricular enlargement. There may be tall P waves and prolongation of the P–R interval.

Treatment   Unlike the ostium secundum defect, surgical correction is much more complicated, often requiring repair of the mitral and tricuspid valves.

Atrio ventricular canal defect

These are virtually an extension of the ostium primum defect which involves the ventricular septum as well. They tend to be more common in children with Down's syndrome.

Clinical manifest-ations   These children tend to present with congestive cardiac failure and recurrent pulmonary infections. On examination the first heart sound may be accentuated and the second heart sound is widely split. There is a loud, harsh pansystolic murmur often associated with a thrill and there is often a low-pitched diastolic murmur audible down the left sternal edge.

Since there is left-to-right shunting at both atrial and ventricular level, pulmonary hypertension can easily occur.

The chest X-ray and e.c.g. findings are similar to those of an ostium primum defect.

Treatment   Surgical correction is complicated and at times banding of the pulmonary artery to reduce pulmonary blood flow is carried out.

Coarctation of the aorta

This is a constriction of the aorta in which about 98% occur just below the origin of the left subclavian artery. The lesion can occur in isolation but is associated with other cardiac abnormalities including bicuspid aortic valve, patent ductus arteriosus and septal defects. Males are more commonly affected than females except those with Turner's syndrome who have an increased incidence.

Heart disease in children

Clinical manifest- ations
A significant proportion of cases are diagnosed on routine examination since symptoms tend to be few in the first decade of life. The symptoms that do occur are due to hypertension giving rise to recurrent epistaxes, headaches and occasionally left ventricular failure. There may be poor circulation in the lower limbs with cold feet occurring with intermittent claudication. Disproportionate body growth with well formed upper limbs and trunk and less well formed lower limbs can occur.

Prompt treatment

Ultrasound
With severe coarctation this may present early in the newborn period with congestive cardiac failure. Early recognition of this condition is important since, if the infant is to survive, not only is prompt medical treatment required of congestive failure, but immediate surgical alleviation of the coarctation before the baby succumbs. Recently ultrasound has been useful in confirming the diagnosis and has avoided the trauma and risk of angiocardiography prior to surgery.

Clinical signs
Clinical signs are classical in the older child, the femoral pulses being either weak and delayed or even absent. If the site of coarctation is above the origin of the subclavian artery, then there will be a diminished left radial pulse as well. On taking blood pressures in the upper and lower limbs there is significant hypertension in the upper limbs. In the normal circulation the popliteal blood pressure is about 20 mmHg above the brachial pressure but this differential is not found in coarctation.

Cardiac murmurs are variable and are not diagnostic and can often be due to associated lesions. The systolic ejection murmur is at times heard at the base of the heart but is often heard maximally at the back in the interscapular region. Bruits and thrills from intercostal vessels are seldom found in young children but may be present in adolescents.

Chest X-rays show a normal or slightly enlarged heart. Rib notching is only evident in later childhood and adolescence. The e.c.g. is either normal or shows left ventricular hypertrophy and occasionally left bundle branch block.

Treatment
Treatment is by surgical resection and this is advisable even if the child is asymptomatic. The optimal age for correction is 3–6 years, depending on the degree of coarctation, mild coarctation sometimes being resected later. In the older child the risk of recoarctation is low while in infancy it still remains significantly high.

Complications
Untreated coarctation of the aorta cases may lead to disparity of growth and hypertension in early adult life which may lead to congestive cardiac failure or cerebral haemorrhage.

77

Transposition of the great vessels

This is a condition where the aorta arises from the right ventricle and the pulmonary artery arises from the left ventricle. The systemic pulmonary veins drain normally. The defect, however, may be associated with other cardiac abnormalities.

Clinical manifestations

These occur early in infancy with central cyanosis and tachypnoea within the first few days of life. Sometimes the onset of cyanosis is delayed due to patency of the foramen ovale and the ductus arteriosus. In a baby who is not obviously suffering from the respiratory distress syndrome, the onset of cyanosis is an indication for immediate cardiac investigation. Delay in referral will only prejudice the prognosis.

The signs on clinical examination are of central cyanosis and tachypnoea. The first heart sound may be accentuated and the second heart sound single or closely split. There is usually no murmur unless there is an additional lesion such as a ventricular septal defect. The liver may be enlarged due to congestive cardiac failure.

The chest X-ray may be normal or the cardiac silhouette may give the 'egg on its side' appearance. The e.c.g. shows normal neonatal right axis deviation and right ventricular hypertrophy but there may, in addition, be P pulmonale.

Treatment

Rashkin's atrial septostomy

Later corrective surgery

Immediate referral to a paediatric cardiothoracic unit is essential because these babies can deteriorate quickly. Having established a diagnosis the atrial septum is ruptured using a balloon catheter, a procedure known as Rashkin's atrial septostomy. This allows venous blood at atrial level to mix and so unsaturated blood can then circulate through the pulmonary circuit. Further corrective surgery is carried out later. For simple transposition, Mustard's procedure involving a baffle, channelling blood from the pulmonary veins to the tricuspid valve, is carried out within the first 2 years of life or, alternatively, a Senning's operation which channels venous blood into the mitral valve. Where there is co-existing pulmonary stenosis and a VSD, if the pulmonary stenosis is severe a shunt procedure is done in order to improve pulmonary circulation. A final operation is then carried out at about the age of 5 using a conduit and valve bypass between the left ventricle and the pulmonary artery and closing the VSD. This is known as the Rastelli procedure. For some appropriate cases switching of the great vessels has been successfully performed.

The prognosis of these complex lesions has greatly improved in recent years, giving a more optimistic outlook for these children but the longterm outlook into adult life is, as yet, to be fully assessed.

Tetralogy of Fallot

This is one of the most commonly recognized cyanotic congenital heart lesions and consists of a combination of the following lesions:

(1) right ventricular outflow obstruction (pulmonary stenosis),
(2) ventricular septal defect,
(3) right ventricular hypertrophy,
(4) overriding (dextroposition) of the aorta.

Cyanosis   Cyanosis is one of the striking features. This may not be present at birth owing to some shunting through the patent ductus arteriosus. As this closes, reducing pulmonary blood flow, so cyanosis begins to appear. Dyspnoea on exertion may occur even in young toddlers and some children may assume the squatting position for relief of dyspnoea after exercise. Cyanotic episodes (blue spells) may be a particular problem in the first 2 years of life. These are due to further reductions in an already impaired pulmonary blood flow giving rise to hypoxia and at times metabolic acidosis. The cyanotic spell may be relieved by:

(1) placing the infant in the prone knee-chest position,
(2) administrating morphine (0.1 mg/kg),
(3) oxygen.

Growth and development in children with this lesion, as with many other severe congenital heart lesions, is often significantly impaired.

Clinical signs   Cyanosis is seen, particularly on exercise or crying, with clubbing of the fingers and toes and secondary polycythaemia. the peripheral pulses are usually normal or diminished. There may be, in infants, a significant precordial bulge. A systolic thrill is palpable in 50% of cases, audible along the left sternal edge. A systolic murmur is audible down the left sternal edge which may be either ejection or pansystolic. In many instances the second heart sound is single.

A chest X-ray shows a concavity of the left heart border due to a diminutive pulmonary conus. The right ventricular border is prominent. The lung fields are oligaemic and the overall picture described as a *coeur en sabot*. The e.c.g. shows right axis deviation and right ventricular hypertrophy. The ultimate diagnosis is confirmed by special investigation including cardiography and cardiac catheterization.

Treatment
Palliative
surgery

Propranolol has been used to alleviate cyanotic attacks until surgery is performed. Surgery is divided into palliative and curative. The main problem is of cyanosis due to inadequate pulmonary blood flow so a shunt operation is often performed at an early stage. These include anastomosis of the subclavian vessel to the pulmonary artery, anastomosis of the aorta to the right pulmonary artery and anastomosis of the descending aorta to the left pulmonary artery. These measures usually produce much improved pulmonary perfusion with the relief of cyanosis and dyspnoea and allow the child to grow and remain in good health until corrective surgery is performed.

Corrective
surgery

Corrective surgery is later performed which involves relieving the pulmonary outflow obstruction and repairing the ventricular septal defect. In suitable cases corrective surgery is carried out in the first instance but overall the two stage procedure is still preferred.

Complications

Owing to the high haematocrit, produced by a secondary polycythaemia, cerebral thrombotic episodes which include cerebral thrombosis and cerebral abscess can occur. It is therefore important to maintain good hydration whenever a child has a high fever or in any situation likely to lead to fluid loss. Prompt and adequate treatment of infection is likewise important.

Pulmonary stenosis

This may either be due to simple valvular stenosis or infundibular stenosis.

Clinical
manifest-
ations

The symptoms are only present usually if the stenosis is severe, causing dyspnoea on effort. Mooned facies are sometimes an associated feature of pulmonary stenosis and it is the commonest cardiac lesion associated with Noonan's syndrome.

The clinical findings on examination are of a loud pulmonary systolic ejection murmur frequently accompanied by a thrill. The murmur is often preceded by a pulmonary systolic ejection click and the pulmonary second sound is split owing to delay of the closure of the pulmonary valve. In infundibular stenosis the murmur often radiates more widely and the ejection click is absent.

The chest X-ray in simple pulmonary stenosis may be normal and the only finding is usually a post-stenotic dilatation of the pulmonary artery. This is usually absent in infundibular stenosis. If the stenosis is severe the right ventricular border may be prominent and the lung fields oligaemic.

The e.c.g. may be normal or show right ventricular hypertrophy and in some instances spiked P waves.

Treatment   Mild cases require no treatment at all but severe pulmonary stenosis will require surgical alleviation.

Aortic stenosis

Congenital valvular stenosis only constitutes about 5% of congenital cardiac lesions in children but it is the commonest lesion found in adults. Males predominate over females and the most common lesion is of the valve itself with thickening of the leaflets and fusion of the commissures. It is often associated with the bicuspid valves.

Facial associations   Simple valvular aortic stenosis can also occur and although rare it is associated with distinct facies comprising a prominent upper lip and a flattened and upturned nose, hypertelorism and is associated with infantile hypercalcaemia.

Subaortic stenosis due to muscular hypertrophy obstructing the left ventricular outflow tract can also occur.

Clinical signs   Mild cases are asymptomatic but severe obstruction can lead to fatigue on exercise, syncope, angina and acute pulmonary oedema. The pulse may be normal or of flow amplitude. A harsh systolic ejection murmur usually accompanied by a thrill is heard in the aortic area radiating to the neck and down the left sternal border. An ejection click usually precedes the murmur in pure aortic stenosis but is absent in supra and subvalvular stenosis. A diastolic murmur may be audible particularly in subaortic stenosis.

The chest X-ray may be normal or show a prominent left ventricle. The ascending aorta may be prominent and occasionally valvular calcification is seen.

The e.c.g. may be normal but if the obstruction is severe left ventricular hypertrophy and strain is seen.

Treatment   Mild cases require treatment at all but surgery is required for those that are symptomatic and have severe obstruction.

Truncus arteriosus

This is a single arterial trunk from the ventricles supplying the systemic pulmonary and coronary circulations. It is always associated with a ventricular septal defect and there are several degrees of the abnormality.

Clinical
features

The clinical picture is similar to a large ventricular septal defect with increased pulmonary blood flow associated with dyspnoea, fatigue, recurrent respiratory tract infection and heart failure.

On examination there is a loud harsh systolic ejection murmur often preceded by a click and the second heart sound is loud and single. A diastolic murmur is audible at the apex and in the axilla.

Chest X-ray shows a large heart, pulmonary plethora. The truncus may produce a distinct bulge and in half the cases this seems to arch to the right.

The e.c.g. shows a variable left and right ventricular hypertrophy.

Treatment

Progress has been made in surgical techniques for treating this condition but it depends on the complexity of the lesion.

Tricuspid atresia

This consists of a hypoplastic right ventricle, a patent foramen ovale, a small ventricular septal defect and often pulmonary artery hypoplasia. Blood therefore flows from the right atrium to the left atrium, and from the left ventricle through the ventricular septal defect into the right ventricle and then into the pulmonary circuit (as well as out through the systemic circulation).

Clinical
manifest-
ations

Cyanosis is a prominent feature, associated with dyspnoea and secondary polycythaemia. In infants a murmur may not be present but usually a pansystolic murmur is audible down the left sternal edge. The pulmonary second sound is absent giving rise to a single second heart sound.

The chest X-ray usually shows pulmonary oligaemia and small pulmonary artery shadows. The right ventricular shadow is diminutive but the left ventricular shadow is prominent.

The e.c.g. characteristically show *left* axis deviation and left ventricular hypertrophy. The P waves may be tall and spiked and in the right sided leads the R wave may be replaced by an RSR complex.

Precautions against infection

Antibiotic
cover

All cases of congenital heart diseases are liable to infective endocarditis and appropriate antibiotic cover should be given for all significant dental procedures, tonsillo-adenoidectomy and all genito-urinary and gastrointestinal surgery. Infective

Infective endocarditis endocarditis should always be considered where there is persistent malaise and fatigue, anaemia and unexplained fever. As infective endocarditis is relatively uncommon and children are prone to many minor infections, the diagnosis can easily be **Dental care** overlooked. Good dental care is a wise precaution in any case, as is the prompt treatment of respiratory tract infection.

7 Metabolic disorders

DIABETES MELLITUS

Clinical manifestations – Stabilization – Insulin – Oral hypogly-caemic agents – Diet – Education – Urine testing – Blood glucose monitoring – Useful services

Incidence

This is a disease which does not spare children and affects about one child in a thousand. It can develop at any age but there tend to be peaks of incidence, the first being at about 5–6 years and the other at puberty. The first peak raises the question of the role of viral illnesses in the aetiology and the second peak the effect of puberty. Childhood diabetes is invariably insulin dependent.

Clinical manifestations

Initial symptoms tend to be of less than 6 weeks duration and sometimes they last only a matter of days. Frequent presenting symptoms are polyuria, nocturia sometimes producing nocturnal

Risk of keto-acidosis

enuresis, polydipsia, weight loss and lethargy. Should infection intervene, the child may present with keto-acidosis giving rise to vomiting, abdominal pain and dehydration. Once the diagnosis has been realized *the child must be referred immediately for stabilization before keto-acidosis intervenes.* Most children with diabetes are best under the care of a paediatrician but in some instances they are under the care of the general physician with a special interest in diabetes. The paediatrician takes a keen interest in diabetes as well as in the problems of children in general.

85

The objectives in the newly diagnosed diabetic child are (1) stabilization and (2) education.

Stabilization

Difficulty in
stabilizing
children

This entails establishing normoglycaemia and estimating the child's insulin requirements. Emphasis on control of diabetes at present is to maintain the diabetic child as near normoglycaemic as possible. Children present particular problems in this respect because of fluctuation in physical activity and irregular eating patterns.

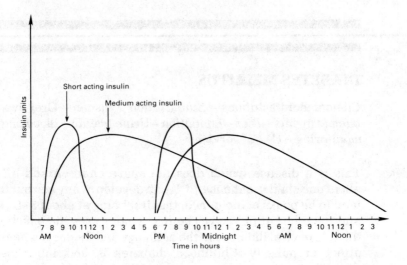

Figure 7.1

Patterns of insulin release

Insulin

Source of
insulin

Monocomponent porcine insulins tend to be preferred these days but it should be emphasized that there is no strong reason for changing a child who is well controlled on bovine insulin.

Insulin regime

In younger children under 5 years old a single daily dose of insulin is adequate but in those children who have unstable diabetes, high insulin requirement and those approaching puberty, twice daily insulin provides better control. A frequently used combination is of a short-acting insulin and medium- or long-acting insulin so as to give a sustained insulin release (Figure 7.1).

There are many insulins on the market at present but on the whole it is better to prescribe those with which one is familiar. There are some children whose needs require a departure from the standard regime so other insulins might be best suited for their needs.

Table 7.1 Spectrum of action of certain insulins

Type	Duration of action (hours)			pH	Source
	Onset	Peak	End		
Short-acting					
Actrapid MC	0.5	3–5	9	7	Porcine
Soluble	1	3–6	8	3	Bovine
Neutral soluble	1	3–6	8	7	Bovine or porcine
Medium-acting					
Semitard	1.5	5–9	15	7	Porcine
Semilente	1.5	5–9	15	7	Bovine or porcine
Ultratard	1.5	4–12	24	7	Porcine
Insulinotard	1.5	4–12	24	7	Porcine
Isophane	2	4–12	24	7	Bovine
Rapitard	1	4–12	22	7	Porcine
Monotard	2	6–14	22	7	Porcine
Long-acting					
Lente	2	6–14	24	7	Bovine or porcine
Protamine zinc	4	10–26	30	7	Bovine

Available strengths

Insulin is currently available in strengths of 20, 40 and 80 units/ml. For the future insulin will be of a universal strength – 100 units/ml. For most children in the past, 40 unit/ml strength insulin has been used. Where insulin requirements have been high 80 units/ml strength has been used in order to reduce the volume of injection.

Adjustment of insulin dosage

Firstly the peaks and troughs of a child's blood sugar levels should be estimated either from scrutinizing the urinalysis charts or, ideally, from blood sugar results. Knowing the length of duration of the insulins prescribed (short-acting or medium-acting) appropriate adjustments can be made. It is important to emphasize that frequent radical changes should not be made otherwise these can produce swings in blood sugar levels giving rise to the somogize effect. A single small adjustment should be made with the aim of avoiding the periods of either hypo- or hyperglycaemia that have been recurring and then estimating the effect of this change in regime over about a week.

Oral hypoglycaemic agents

The question of their use is often raised by parents in the hope that their child will not require injections. In fact, the evidence to date shows that they have no place in the treatment of juvenile diabetes. There are recorded instances of a few children with minimal insulin requirements who have been controlled by oral hypoglycaemic agents but they are very rare.

Diet

Opinions have fluctuated over the question of dietary control. There have been advocates of tight and liberal control and in reality it is not possible to get children to conform. A danger of excessive tight control is that children can remain small and stunted through lack of dietary intake and also miserable due to subclinical hypoglycaemia. A too liberal approach, however, can lead to excessive hyperglycaemia and prematurely to the complications of the longterm diabetic. A controlled carbohydrate diet is the most commonly used. Among the formulae used to calculate the daily carbohydrate need is

Limited carbohydrate diet

$$(100) + [10 \times \text{age in years}] = \text{daily requirement in grams}$$

e.g. a 4-year-old girl gets 140 g of carbohydrate a day increasing in adolescence up to about 220 g a day.

Protein and fat

Very young children

High fibre diet

Protein and fat are unregulated. In the very young child it is often difficult to specifically restrict carbohydrate and so an initial free diet can be used but obviously excluding free sugar, jam and sweets. At present a high fibre diet is advocated since there is some evidence to show that on such a diet the blood sugar level rises more steadily, producing less hyperglycaemia.

It is helpful to utilize the services of a dietitian who can discuss with the parents and the child a diet and tailor it to accommodate his existing eating habits as well as his daily needs.

Education

Few diseases require such extensive education of the parents and patient as diabetes. Initial education is the most important of all. It is very difficult to reform a non-conforming diabetic and poorly controlled childhood diabetics seldom reform in adult life. A step-by-step education of the parents (and the child if old enough to understand) is very important. Explanations should be plain and simple. The full nature of diabetes, its method of control, problems and complications should be explained. In the majority of instances the better the parents' knowledge of the disease, the more able both they and the child are to use this knowledge in order to maintain good control. This does, of course, beg the question as to what is good control. This should incorporate the following.

Good diabetic control

(1) The child is healthy, active and enjoying life.
(2) Growth is satisfactory. Several studies have been performed and it is found overall that the growth of diabetic children is less than predicted had they not had diabetes. However, any gross lag of growth beyond this expectation is indicative of poor control. For this reason it is essential to keep a growth chart (Tanner and Whitehouse) in order to chart growth.
(3) Urine tests, although they are subject to inaccuracy, should ideally only show a trace of sugar occasionally and no ketones.
(4) There should be no hypo- or hyperglycaemia and the blood glucose levels should be within the 3–10 mmol/l range making allowances for the time of day and meal-times.

Results of poor control

It should be stressed that lax control may not only lead to keto-acidosis but to sub-optimal health, impaired growth and early diabetic complications, particularly diabetic retinopathy and probably the other recognized complications as well. On the other hand, obsessive control can give rise to impaired growth from dietary restriction, hypoglycaemia which may be sub-clinical giving rise to general malaise and possibly rebellious problems in adolescence. Common sense must prevail with both the physician and patient in order to achieve good control without undue restriction.

Result of obsessive control

Diet

The full implications of the dietary measures should be explained and this requires an explanation of the fundamental constituents of food and the appropriate calorific values. The help of the dietitian can be most valuable in this respect. Often advice on matters such as holiday and travel are important and also adjustment of diet to deal with special circumstances such as taking extra calories prior to planned physical activities in order to avoid hypoglycaemia.

Special circumstances

Insulin

Explanation of the mode of action of insulin and the onset and duration of its action are most important. Likewise, it is important to explain the varying strengths of insulin prepar-

Dosage

ations, since this is a source of potential confusion (hopefully this will be eliminated with the use of the new 100 unit/ml standardization). Insulin should be kept between 4 and 10 °C in order to maintain its potency. Instructions on drawing up insulin and how to mix insulins without contamination are important.

Storage

Injections

The types of syringe and how to give the injection (including sites of injection) are important and must be explained. It is quite common to find that diabetics who are requiring increasing amounts of insulin are injecting repeatedly into one site which has become hard and sclerematous with subsequent poor absorption of insulin.

Self-injections

Educating the child to give his own injections at the earliest reasonable opportunity is very important. Ages of reaching competence to achieve this vary but by the age of 10–12 years most children manage most of the time. There is a tendency for some parents to continue giving the injections so that the children become dependent on them and it is necessary to teach these children to give their own injections so they can become independent of their parents in managing their own diabetes.

Syringe guns

There are some children who resist their injections and for some of these the syringe gun can be useful (syringe guns can be obtained from either Palmer Injectors Ltd., PO Box 10, Vulcan Works, Paisley, PA3 4BE, Scotland, or from Hypoguard Ltd., 14 Second Avenue, Trimley, Ipswich, Suffolk). Disposable

Syringe needles

syringe needles are less traumatic and the short 25G are the most suitable. They can be used at least 3–4 times if used carefully and are best kept in industrial methylated spirits (rather

Disposable syringes

than surgical spirit which tends to be greasy). Disposable syringes are preferred by some and likewise these can be preserved in spirit. It should be remembered that disposable syringes and needles can only be prescribed under the NHS under special circumstances requiring a hospital consultant's backing. This should provide no difficulty if the need is real. Otherwise the standard insulin syringe is prescribed, BS 1619, which may be 1 or 2 ml in size and is graduated in 20 units/ml.

Urine testing

This aspect of diabetic management is subject to much abuse and misinterpretation by the physician. When should the urine tests be done and for what? Once the patient is stabilized twice-daily testing, before breakfast and before the evening meal, is sufficient. However, prior to full stabilization or at times when there is subsequent instability, testing four times a day is essential (before breakfast, lunch, supper and before bedtime) in order to see the spectrum of control. In any case it is a good idea about once a week to test the urine four times a day just to see that control is satisfactory overall. Particularly with the early morning specimen, double micturition is important if the child is old enough to co-operate in order to obtain a result more relevant to that time. Testing the urine for sugar with Clinistix involves adhering to a strict procedure if the results are to be valid.

Double micturition

Clinistix

(1) The test tube and dropper should be *dry*.
(2) Only the dropper supplied with the set should be used and the dropper should be held vertically over the tube when the drops are released.
(3) Having measured 5 drops of the urine into the test tube, the dropper should be rinsed before taking up the water.
(4) Once the tablet has been added, the complete reaction must be watched in order not to miss a transient orange colour due to high sugar content.
(5) The equipment must be washed and dried completely after usage.

Ketodiastix can be used as an alternative particularly when out for the day when it is inconvenient to test urine in the normal manner. They have the advantage of convenience but do have the disadvantage of requiring a precise reaction time.

Testing for ketones

Testing for ketones is very important when diabetes is unstable and there is excessive glycosuria. It may be very important at times of infection. During good health otherwise there is no indication for routine testing.

'Dishonesty' over testing

While errors can occur due to poor technique of testing, the most important of all is that the patient is honest about his tests. A rather tattered chart indicates that it is well used while the chart that is very meticulous can be indicative that it was made up just prior to seeing a doctor. Often much hinges on the urine results and so it is important to try and ascertain if they are genuine, otherwise an inappropriate change of insulin dosage can be made.

Blood glucose monitoring at home

In the past few years there has been a series of blood glucose monitors appearing on the market. There seems some logic in their use as they monitor directly the blood glucose level with relative ease so the spectrum of results can be obtained without all the difficulties of resorting to the hospital laboratory. As with most ventures, it tends to fall into perspective once the initial wave of enthusiasm settles. Used sensibly and correctly these instruments are very useful in the good control of diabetes. The

Advantages main advantages are that the spectrum of blood glucose levels can be done periodically (once or twice a week) to see that the patient is normoglycaemic and that the results coincide with the urine tests. At times of problems it is particularly useful to see if the diabetic is either hypo- or hyperglycaemic. The disadvant-

Disadvantages ages are seen if there is poor technique in estimating the blood sugar, poor motivation and little heed is taken of the result. At the other end of the spectrum, excessive zeal may result in the child having undue finger pricks and life being centred on the results from the machine.

In order to use the monitors to advantage, parents must appreciate the normal fluctuations in blood glucose. From their results the sensible parent and child are able to make the appropriate adjustments in the insulin according to the results. Some parents are prepared to buy a blood glucose monitor outright while for others periodic loan might be better.

Monitors in
surgeries
It would seem useful for most family doctors' surgeries to be equipped with a blood glucose monitor as it affords an easy spot check on diabetics and could be most useful on emergency calls to the diabetic with unstable control.

Useful services

British
Diabetic
Association
The British Diabetic Association through its local branches provides invaluable support to diabetic families through meetings, leaflets and personal communication. In addition, there are many other activities including the summer diabetic camp which most children enjoy and find very beneficial.

Community
Nursing Sister
Many Districts now have a Community Nursing Sister who visits the diabetics at home and checks their progress and advises accordingly and she, in turn, reports back to both the family doctor and the hospital consultant. This has proved a valuable way of seeing diabetics at home as they really are, and many parents and children find it easier to approach the nurse on aspects that they are worried about rather than the doctor in a busy clinic.

Social care
In some families the strain of knowing that they have got a diabetic child, especially where there are pre-existing difficulties, justify the help of a social worker in order to see them through.

There is a lot at stake with the juvenile diabetic and it behoves us all to provide optimal care, not only for their health at present, but for their longterm health in the future.

THYROID DISORDERS

Thyrotoxicosis – Carcinoma of the thyroid – Hypothyroidism

Thyrotoxicosis

Aetiology In most instances this is due to Graves disease, a diffuse toxic goitre. It is thought that immune factors are involved in the pathogenesis especially since thyroid enlargement, splenomegaly and lymphadenopathy are associated features. An immunoglobulin is produced which binds to the receptor for TSH and at the same time stimulates the process normally set in motion by TSH. A number of antibodies can be demonstrated including LATS (long-acting thyroid stimulator).

Table 7.2 Normal serum levels of tri-iodothyronine (T_4) and thyroid stimulating hormone (TSH)

	Thyroxine (T_4) (nmol/l)	TSH (mU/ml)
0–24 hours	178–330	3–120
1 week +	154–265	<1–10
4 weeks–1 year	90–195	<1–5
1 year–10 years	70–180	<1–5

Table 7.3 Thyroxine dosage according to age

2 months–1 year	12.5 µg daily	
1–7 years	25 µg daily	} according to responses
7–14 years	50 µg daily	

Most cases occur in adolescence and girls are more commonly affected than boys (very occasionally the disease can occur in the neonatal period). Symptoms usually develop over 6–12 months and may present with emotional disturbances and motor hyperexcitability in addition to the other signs. The thyroid is diffusely enlarged. Growth is often accelerated although subsequent development is not altered.

Clinical suspicions are confirmed by thyroid function tests. The thyroxine (T_4) and tri-iodothyronine (T_3) levels are increased and the thyroid stimulating hormone (TSH) is low (Table 7.2).

Medical treatment
Propylthiouracil or carbimazole are the drugs of choice. Propylthiouracil has the additional advantage of inhibiting peripheral conversion of T_4 to T_3.

Propranolol counteracts troublesome symptoms such as tachycardia but has no other effect.

Antithyroid treatment with drugs is needed for at least 2 years before withdrawal of therapy, symptoms usually remitting in the majority of children. Careful follow-up after cessation of therapy is required to detect either relapse or progression to hypothyroidism.

Surgical treatment
Subtotal thyroidectomy has no strong indications in childhood but if medical treatment fails, then it is the next step.

Radioactive iodine
There is no indication for radioactive iodine in children.

Carcinoma of the thyroid

This is rare in children but must be considered in the differential diagnosis of goitre. Papillary carcinoma is the more common histological type and tends to be more malignant with advancing age.

Hypothyroidism

Infantile hypo-thyroidism
The incidence of congenital hypothyroidism is in the order of 1 in 4000 live births. There is a fallacy in placing reliance on clinical features because some babies who appear to look like cretins are quite normal and others who appear normal have proven hypothyroidism. In addition, when there are obvious clear-cut features of hypothyroidism, this is usually at a late stage in the diagnosis and the prognosis after treatment is less favourable.

The implications of disordered thyroid function are immense because of the devastating effect of hypothyroidism on brain development. Neonatal screening programmes are now underway in many regions since the need for these is really greater than that for screening for phenylketonuria. In the light of the implications of hypothyroidism tests must be carried out when there is the slightest suggestion on clinical and developmental grounds that the disorder may be present. These include

94

failure to thrive, delay in achieving developmental milestones and prolonged neonatal jaundice not attributed to other causes.

Diagnosis

This ultimately entirely depends on laboratory data. The serum thyroxine (T_4) is low and the TSH levels significantly elevated. If the TSH is not low (i.e. not primary hypothyroidism) a TRH (thyroid releasing hormone test) is required to see the response of TSH in cases due to hypopituitism.

Responses vary from patient to patient and it is important to continue monitoring thyroid function along with growth. It must be explained to the parents that excessive dosage is harmful and being a deficiency state 'the more the better' is an inappropriate philosophy. (Table 7.2).

Presentation later in childhood

While thyroid dysgenesis almost invariably presents early in infancy, there are some cases that can present later. Growth retardation is one manifestation and it may not be apparent for some time until the child appears obviously smaller than his peers. Hence routine measurement of height for all school children is important since it may be an easy way of spotting the child with previously undiagnosed hypothyroidism.

Enzyme deficiencies

Enzyme deficiencies are uncommon and usually present with asymptomatic goitres. Iodine deficiency is very rare.

Auto-immune thyroid disease

Auto-immune thyroid disease may present as hypo- or hyperthyroidism. These cases tend to present in adolescence. It can be associated with other diseases which include diabetes mellitus and adrenal cortical insufficiency.

Hypothalamo-pituitary axis disorders constitute the commonest cause other than those due to thyroid hypoplasia or aplasia.

Treatment with thyroxine

Thyroxine (0.1 mg per square metre of the body surface area per day) is the standard treatment regime but the response in individuals varies. As with infants, careful monitoring of growth and thyroid function tests are important. It is usually found that after retardation of growth there is a period of catch-up once treatment is started and then the child should proceed along the expected centile. Again, excessive dosage should be avoided as this advances the bone age, producing premature fusion of the epiphyses with ultimate shortness of stature. It is therefore counterproductive in producing normal growth.

CONGENITAL ADRENAL HYPERPLASIA

This is a condition with an incidence of 1 in 5000 live births. The

Clinical
features

most common enzyme pathway deficiency is the 21-hydroxylase deficiency. The important features of this disorder are:

(1) ambiguous genitalia in the female,
(2) salt-losing crisis,
(3) precocious puberty,
(4) family history of congenital adrenal hypoplasia or unexplained neonatal death,
(5) hirsuitism and signs of mascularization in the mature female and
(6) Males with cryptochordism whose genotype is female.

Diagnosis

The diagnosis is confirmed by finding elevated levels of 17-oxosteroids in a 24-hour urine sample or elevated 17-hydroxyprogesterone levels in the blood.

Treatment

Treatment is with longterm mineralo- and glucocorticoid replacement. Hydrocortisone 20 mg per square metre of body surface area per 24 hours is often used but it is a matter of individual preference as to which steroid is used.

Importance in longterm management is that the replacement therapy is adequate and this is checked by urinary 17-oxosteroid levels or plasma 17-hydroxyprogesterone levels or ACTH levels. As with thyroid disorders it is important to monitor growth with bone age.

GROWTH PROBLEMS

Short stature – Differential diagnosis of short stature – Tall children

Short stature

Normal short
stature

There is frequent concern about short stature and in fact the majority of children thought to be short are quite normal and constitute the 3% of children whose stature is below the third percentile. These children usually have short parents. The

Growth
velocity

growth velocity is a means of distinguishing the short but normal child from those who are pathologically short. It is therefore

Accurate
height
measurement

important to measure the height of children accurately and record it on a chart (Tanner and Whitehouse height and weight charts). To do this the child must stand erect and the head must be held with the external auditory meatus and the outer angle of the eye in a horizontal plane. Pressure is applied under the mastoid process to encourage the child to stretch upwards in order to eliminate changes in posture. It is vitally important that the procedure is adhered to and that the same person, if possible, measures the child. Measurements at random by untrained staff are worthless and under these circumstances I have even seen a child measured with their shoes on! The accuracy of the measuring apparatus is equally important. The Harpenden stadiometer is one of such instruments capable of giving accurate measurement. The single measurement of a child's height is not adequate since the child whose height is below the third percentile may be quite normal, whereas another whose height is on the 50th centile may require investigation, hence growth velocity measurement is all important. This requires two measurements of height over a period of at least 3 months, or better, over 12 months. Growth velocity is the incremental rise in stature between two measurements divided by the time interval. If height velocity is less than the 50th centile for any length of time, short stature will ensue.

Expected height
In order to roughly calculate expected height, for a boy the father's height is plotted on the centile chart and the mother's height plus 12.5 cm. The mid-point between the father's height and the mother plus 12.5 cm gives the expected 50th centile for that family. For a girl the mother's height is plotted and 12.5 cm deducted from the father's height, giving the 50th centile for girls of that family.

Differential diagnosis of short stature

The following considerations can be made in the differential diagnosis of short stature*:

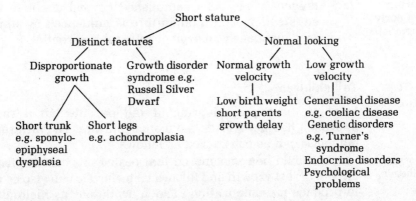

*Adapted from Brook C. G. D., Practical Paediatric Endocrinology 1978

Certain aspects are worthy of note.

Normal small stature and growth delay

(1) Proportionately short children – this is where growth velocity measurements are important because the child who has had low growth velocity requires a diagnosis and treatment. Some children are smaller but grow normally, having been born of low birthweight or of small parents or whose span of growth is longer than most children. Some children enter puberty later and continue to grow late. These children have proportionate delay in bone age which may also occur in some endocrine disorders. However, provided that the growth velocity is normal there is no need for further investigation.

Coeliac disease

(2) Coeliac disease can present in many guises and solitary lack of growth can, on occasions, be the only feature. Jejunal biopsy is the only satisfactory way of proving the diagnosis.

Social deprivation

(3) Profound social deprivation, which may or may not include starvation, should always be considered when other causes are not evident.

Hypo-thyroidism

(4) Hypothyroidism is always an important endocrine cause to consider.

Turner's syndrome

(5) In the short female Turner's syndrome must always be excluded.

Growth hormone deficiency

Importance of early recognition

(6) Children with human growth hormone deficiency are characterized by shortness of stature and are usually well nourished. Growth hormone is only prescribed on approval of certain designated MRC centres once the diagnosis has been established beyond doubt to their satisfaction. The final stature is influenced by starting treatment early so prompt referral is essential.

Tall children

Most of these are offspring of tall parents but a similar approach has to be made as in short stature. The differential diagnosis can be considered as follows.

Hormone therapy

It should be remembered that oestrogens can be given to girls to arrest growth and in boys testosterone can also be used to produce masculinization in such conditions as Kleinfelter's syndrome.

Metabolic disorders

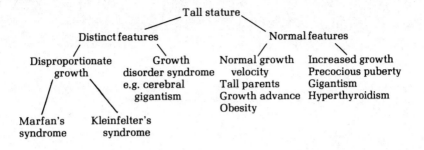

⑧ Common symptoms and problems of doubtful origin

Abdominal pain – Headaches – Nocturnal enuresis – Faecal soiling and encopresis

There are many children who are brought to their family doctor or to the hospital with symptoms and problems not due to primary organic disease. There is often considerable anxiety about these and sometimes they are brought with parental demands that 'something must be done'. Among these symptoms include the following.

Abdominal pain

This is a common symptom in young children and because of the implications that there might be some intra-abdominal pathology, parents are usually quite swift to seek advice and rightly so. The most important action is to take a detailed history of the child's symptoms as well as a family history as this may be relevant, followed by physical examination (rectal examination is usually not included unless there are special indications). Examination of the urine, however, is important in case of urinary tract infection.

Abdominal pain in the peri-umbilical region has a lesser likelihood of being due to an organic cause than to pain elsewhere. Having come to the conclusion that there is unlikely to be any serious intra-abdominal pathology, the most important part of the consultation is to carefully explain to the parents the whole background of abdominal pain in childhood and that having carefully examined the child there is nothing to suggest any organic ailment.

Detailed history

Explanation to parents

101

Up to 1 in 10 of children suffer from recurrent abdominal pain for which there are no obvious specific causes. It tends to peak at certain ages, 4–5 years in both sexes and again in the pre-adolescent period in girls. The family history may well be relevant as there seems quite a significant association between migraine and dyspepsia in the parents and the child who suffers from recurrent abdominal pain and the so-called irritable bowel syndrome. As the late John Apley quoted, 'little bellyachers often grow into big bellyachers'. It is of interest too that many such children with recurrent abdominal pain later develop migraine and it is not suprising as the pathologies of both are similar.

Association with migraine

Explaining to the parents the details of the situation is often sufficient to put their minds at rest and the tensions around the child's symptoms become less, to the extent that they accept that it is all part of the difficulties of growing up. Investigations are best avoided apart from urinalysis, since they tend only to perpetuate the parents' fears of some underlying serious organic problem. At times a full blood count, chest X-ray and abdominal X-ray are performed to satisfy the parents but it is rarely necessary to embark upon barium studies, intravenous pyelograms or anything else unless there are other specific indications to do so.

Investigations

While abdominal pains are common and usually innocent in nature, all children can develop acute appendicitis. In this respect it should be mentioned to the parents that should there be any change in the nature of the pain or there be any other associated symptoms, then immediate medical advice should be sought.

Risk of appendicitis

The child with the abdominal pain due to non-organic causes is as distressed as a child who has definite organic disease. Paracetamol may be quite effective in alleviating symptoms as may antispasmodics such as dicyclomine. For the child who may well have abdominal migraine a trial of Bellergal (belladonna, ergotamine and phenobarbitone) may well be effective. Overall reassurance is the most important measure but otherwise medication should be kept to the minimum necessary to alleviate symptoms.

Treatment

Drugs

Headaches

Many aspects of headaches in children bear semblance to the problem of recurrent abdominal pain and the approach is

Detailed history

Character of headache
Examination

similar. A medical history including family and social conditions is important in order to obtain the socio-medical background. Examination should include neurological examination, looking for signs of raised intracranial pressure and ataxia. Measurement of head circumference and blood pressure are vital. Many parents fear that their child may have a cerebral tumour or some other malignant condition. It should be remembered that recurrent headache tends to be uncommon before the age of 5 years. If the headache is occipital rather than frontal and occurs more in the mornings than the evenings and is associated with vomiting, then it is more likely to be due to an organic cause.

Ominous signs

In children ominous signs of intracranial lesion include ataxia, papilloedema, enlarged head with a boxy percussion note. Examination of the optic fundi in children is not as difficult as is made out and many children will co-operate almost as well as adults. Although cerebral tumours are rare in children, the diagnosis is often made late which often reduces the prognosis.

Investigations

Further investigation is not required if the history and examination are entirely normal. If symptoms persist, a skull X-ray and full blood count are justified and an ophthalmic opinion is sometimes helpful in a child who has a refractive error. A feature of non-organic headache is that it is usually fleeting and the child will carry on playing, often saying that the headache lasted for only a few minutes. Other children, however, may look depressed and unhappy and this might be suggestive of family or school problems.

Careful discussion with the parents and child is very important to put both their minds at rest. It is important to follow these children up to see that no other symptoms develop and if there is on-going difficulty referral to the local paediatrician is advised. Sadly, there are too many children who have had cerebral tumours which have gone undiagnosed for too long because their persisting symptoms and signs have gone unnoticed.

Risk of undiagnosed cerebral tumour

Treatment

Medication

The aim of management is in putting the family's mind at rest. Fleeting headaches require no treatment at all but for those that are more persistent paracetamol or soluble aspirin may be recommended. There are those children who undoubtedly suffer from migraine and a combination of soluble aspirin and metoclopramide is often effective in reducing the nausea as well as the pain. For the older child ergotamine compounds can be used and for the chronic migraine sufferer Catapres (Dixarit) or propranolol can be tried on a longterm prophylactic basis with variable success. On the whole, longterm medication is best

Diet   avoided except for the child with the recurrent symptoms. Dietary considerations are also relevant in migraine, avoiding chocolate, cheese and citrus fruits is thought to possibly reduce the frequency of attacks. Recording of attacks by parents in a diary may be helpful in indicating effectiveness of therapy.

Recording attacks

Nocturnal enuresis

Incidence   A very common referral to out-patients but rather an unnecessary one. Children vary in the age at which they gain nocturnal continence of urine. About 10–15% of normal children at the age of 5 years and about 1% at the age of 15 years still wet the bed at night. Boys slightly predominate over girls and there is an increased incidence in some families. One is therefore going to accept that nocturnal enuresis is not significantly abnormal up to the age of 5–6 years. The factors leading to gaining bladder control are complex and involve maturation of the necessary neurological pathways as well as emotional factors.

Features which are important to take note of are the following.

Relapse to enuresis

(1) The child who has previously been continent who becomes enuretic again. This may be due to organic disease including urinary tract infection, diabetes mellitus or insipidus or any other illness or condition. Alternatively, there may be emotional factors which have caused the child's regress.

Day-time enuresis

(2) The occurrence with day-time enuresis is particularly significant and may be related to urinary tract infection or diabetes mellitus.

Detailed history

The matter is approached in the usual manner of noting specific details of the child's urinary symptomatology and the family history. It is not so uncommon to encounter parents who are indignant that their 4-year-old still wets the bed, yet they themselves were not dry until the age of 15. A physical examination is made including examination of the abdomen, genitalia, spine and careful neurological examination below the waistline. Examination of the urine for protein, sugar, microscopical examination and culture are mandatory.

Examination

For the vast majority of children the history dates from infancy, the enuresis is entirely nocturnal, physical examination is normal and the urine is clear. In these circumstances further investigations, such as IVP and micturating cystogram, are not required unless there is additional indication such as a history of urinary tract infection.

Management
    In the management of nocturnal enuresis, the significant actions are as follows.

Explanation
(1) It is important to carefully explain to the parents the nature and course of nocturnal enuresis and that all children in the course of time will become continent of urine. This is important to explain to the child as well, as he may feel that he never will be dry at night.

Avoid full bladder at bedtime
(2) Emptying the bladder before going to bed and lifting the child before the parents go to bed often helps Avoiding excessive fluid intake before bedtime might be helpful but it should be remembered that children require a relatively higher fluid intake than adults and so fluids before bedtime can only be restricted within reason.

Star chart
(3) A star chart and giving plenty of praise for a dry night is a good incentive. Nagging and punishment are usually counterproductive.

Medication
(4) The tricyclic drugs, imipramine and amitriptyline, for the child over 6 years can often help. The dosage for the child under 8 years is 25 mg, over 8 years 50 mg and over 10 years 75 mg *nocte* are used. For many children it will establish a pattern and boost morale. Some, however, may relapse when the drug is stopped and relapse is less frequent when the drug is withdrawn slowly. A course of at least 6 weeks is usually required.

Enuresis alarm
(5) The enuresis alarm is probably a safe and effective method, providing there is co-operation of both parent and child. It usually takes 3–4 weeks before treatment begins to be effective and so it should therefore be tried for at least 6 weeks to see if it is going to work.

Organic conditions
(6) For those children with organic conditions their symptoms resolve on controlling the organic condition. In those children with profound emotional problems, at times the opinion of the child psychiatrist may well be helpful.

Desmopressin
(7) There are some indications in the older child for using DDAVP (desmopressin) but this should only be done under hospital supervision, when all other methods have failed.

Faecal soiling and encopresis

Background causes
This is quite a common condition, its causes are complex and its treatment prolonged and tedious. The background causes include the following.

105

(1) The child who becomes fluid-depleted, often due to febrile illness and becomes constipated, producing rock-hard faeces. When defaecation eventually occurs, evacuation of the bowel produces a tear in the anal sphincter giving rise to a painful fissure. Thereafter the child is very reluctant to have his bowels open.
(2) The child with neglected toilet training.
(3) The child whose parents have been obsessive about toilet training from an early age.
(4) The emotionally deprived child, who fails to use the toilet and soils probably as a mode of expressing his emotional demands.

Examination   Many of these children on examination are found to have a large faecal mass palpable per abdomen. On rectal examination faeces are often found between the glutei and the anal sphincter is usually dilated and patulous and the rectum full of a solid faecal core. These children seldom seem distressed at rectal examination. The fact that the rectum is loaded with faeces is useful in differentiating from Hirschsprung's disease, where the rectum is usually empty.

Effects   The effects of chronic constipation are the following.

(1) Distension of the colon and rectum so that normal muscular ability to evacuate the colon is lost.
(2) Gross distension of the rectum and anal canal leads to loss of the normal sensation of an urge to defaecate and so the child is no longer aware of when he is faecally incontinent.
(3) The huge faecal core tends to liquify on the outside and the fluid content of the bowel oozes out at the anus. At times this is wrongly interpreted as diarrhoea and inappropriate medication prescribed.

Treatment

Enemas   The first aim of treatment is to empty the bowel but it is best to avoid enemas, washouts and suppositories unless other Faecal measures fail. The use of faecal softening agents coupled with softeners aperients works effectively in a high proportion of cases. Among the medications that can be used are lactulose and Diocytyl-Medo. Methylcellulose compounds are also useful but many Purgatives children find them unpalatable. Use of purgatives is contro-versial but it is reasonable to use such preparations as Senokot until the bowel is emptied and normal bowel action is established. Due to the longterm effects of prolonged purgative use, this should be withdrawn as soon as is reasonably possible.

Painful fissure
For the child with the painful fissure appropriate local analgesic ointment can be applied before defaecation in addition to faecal softening agents in order to make defaecation less painful.

Dietary measures
Dietary measures are also important and these include a good fluid intake. Encouragement to take an adequate amount of roughage in the diet is likewise important as many of these children tend to prefer a low residue diet.

Regular toileting
Regular toileting, daily after mealtimes, is important in order to set up a regular habit of defaecation.

Psychological factors
In most children with faecal soiling and encopresis there are strong psychological factors behind the problem. The help of a child psychiatrist may help in eliciting the fundamental cause and directing therapy. In practice, one often tends to refer such children where obvious emotional factors prevail and also those whose progress has been slow.

Hospital admission
While the majority of children can be treated at home, there are some children where fundamental measures fail and so admission to hospital is needed for enemas and toilet training.

Longterm approach
Patience and tolerance to persevere with the problem over many months and, if necessary years, are very important. This is not so much dealing with the child as dealing with the pressures from the parents. Reassurance that in spite of the longevity of the problem, it will eventually resolve, is important. Rarely do incontinent children become incontinent adults.

Encopresis

This is a problem of faecal soiling and defaecation in inappropriate places. It can be coupled with the problem of faecal soiling. In these children the rectum is empty. The background to this is inevitably psychological and almost always requires the assistance of a child psychiatrist. Admission to hospital is sometimes useful in some children. For those children who smear faeces, regular toileting and the use of bowel softening agents so that the rectum is empty, is sometimes helpful in reducing the extent of smearing.

Psychological background

The problem child

The crying baby – Breath-holding attacks – Temper tantrums – The overactive child – The child who does not sleep – The child who does not eat – School problems

There are nearly as many occasions that a child is brought to the doctor because of behaviour problems or difficulties as for acute illness. Unlike acute illness, in which there is usually a simple clear-cut cause and treatment, behavioural problems require time, patience and understanding to sort out. Some of these problems are discussed below.

The crying baby

All babies cry, some are placid and happy babies and others are not so contented. Beyond the range of normal there are babies who cry nearly all the time and particularly at night. As in all situations a clinical evaluation is essential to exclude rare but serious organic conditions such as intussusception, strangulated hernia, otitis media or even acute osteitis or arthritis. Injury is important to consider as well. Poor feeding techniques, or even the possibility of cow's milk protein intolerance giving rise to gastrointestinal colic. Having carefully considered all possibilities, one is often left with a screaming and desperate baby and tired and very fraught parents. It is often difficult to see when the trouble began because crying babies upset parents and upset parents further upset babies and it all becomes a vicious circle. In many instances it is important to realize that there may be a problem of initial bonding. The baby who is aware that he is emotionally rejected can become very irritable

Exclusion of organic conditions and injury

Poor feeding techniques

Gastrointestinal colic

Problem of initial bonding

and cry incessantly. In the hands of a mother who has no great feeling for the baby, he is very much at risk to non-accidental injury. Likewise, the insecure mother who senses her anxiety may also get to the point of loss of control after a prolonged period of enduring the screaming baby and lack of sleep. In both instances it is important to be prepared to spend time in order to get to the bottom of things.

Hospital admission

Social services

At times, to pack the baby off to a helpful friend or relative is fully justified or even admission to hospital in order to allow the parents a chance to sleep and regain their composure. In the case of the overwrought mother it is important to give reassurance and continued support to see her over the difficulty. For the child who is rejected, it is wise to enlist the help of a health visitor or social worker and, where necessary, to convene a case conference in order to inform all workers involved of the problem. It is foolhardy to fail to heed the early signs of rejection when early help can avert a disaster.

Breath-holding attacks

This is a phenomenon of the first 3 years of life and starts at about 6 months of age. The child, when he is upset, will hold his breath to the point of becoming cyanosed. Very rarely such a child will hold his breath long enough to produce an anoxic fit.

Management

The correct management is to ignore the whole episode as fussing the child tends to perpetuate the attack. Mild sedation has been advocated in the past but overall has little influence.

Careful explanation to parents

Breath-holding attacks have to be considered in the differential diagnosis of epilepsy and parents may question as to whether the child suffers from cyanotic congenital heart disease. A careful explanation of the attacks, their management and the outlook should be given to the parents who are then in a much better position to cope, in the knowledge that the attacks are harmless and self-limiting.

Temper tantrums

Uncontrollable anger

These tend to predominate in the 2–4 year age group when the child develops aggression and anger but has yet to learn to control it. All children show anger and it is only the child with uncontrollable anger who is the real problem. Before expecting the child to control his anger, it is important to tactfully elicit whether the parents can control theirs, as such a parent is

110

unlikely to be effective in controlling the anger of their own child. Many tantrums are caused by the intelligent child who has limited language to express himself and such children improve rapidly when they can make their grievances known.

Importance of avoiding confrontation

It is important to advise parents to avoid confrontation where possible, either ignoring the tantrums so that the child receives little attention from it or distracting the child, which is often the greatest adult weapon in dealing with a difficult child. Children of this age group have a fairly brief attention span and a sensible parent is able to easily distract them from whatever induced the rage. By this one does not imply that children should have their own way but where possible they should be distracted from their tantrum and subsequently encouraged to control their temper and given praise when they show signs of achieving this.

Distracting the angry child

The overactive child

Risk of overdiagnosis

The hyperactive child is over-diagnosed and it should be realized that healthy children are usually very active and busy people. However, there are children who are active beyond normal bounds. Overactivity is inevitably accompanied by a very short attention span, sometimes delay in learning and usually other behavioural difficulties as well. In many instances a careful history will reveal emotional conflict at some stage, eiher the mother had anxieties in pregnancy or bonding with the newborn baby was poor and maybe the child is not the product of a planned pregnancy. So often the emotional problems of the child are a manifestation of parental rejection at the outset.

Behavioural difficulties

Emotional problems

Mental retardment

Dietary causes

There are many children in whom there is no obvious background cause. In some instances the mentally retarded child may present in this manner. There are some children in whom some dietary elements may be a causative factor. Evidence for this is difficult to prove but many of these children do seem to improve on the Feingold diet and for this reason it is worth a trial. Similarly it is important to check that the child is not receiving medication that may cause hyperactivity such as anticonvulsants, particularly phenobarbitone.

Feingold diet

Medication as a cause

Advice to the parents

Advising the parents is important. Many do not spend very much time talking and playing with their children. Some homes are devoid of sensible toys and the facilities to play. The child in the immaculate home is just at much at risk as the child in a hovel. Getting the child to settle and play with something he likes in order to cultivate concentration is important, not only from the behavioural aspect, but to enable him to concentrate and learn. Medication seldom helps with such children but early placement in a well-structured play group, may not only help the child but will also enable the parents to have some respite.

The child who does not sleep

Babies who do not settle at night and children who will not sleep are common problems and often solutions are difficult to provide. They will in the course of time spontaneously resolve but this is of little consolation to the desperate parents. Of course newborn babies wake at night for their feed and some will remain awake. It is important to examine the baby in case of conditions such as otitis media which may be causing the baby to be fretful. The advice of feeding and settling the baby for bed in a quiet and orderly manner and then leaving the baby undisturbed for as long as possible without rushing to attend to him, is easily given but not so easily heeded. The crying baby left for a while will not come to any harm and, to a certain extent, those babies that are picked up most readily are those that wake and cry most often.

Chloral hydrate (30 mg/kg body weight) can be used to settle the baby who cries incessantly at night. Its effect is often only transient and so it is best used for a few nights at a time in order to give the parents some respite. If the baby has cried incessantly it may be necessary to admit the baby to hospital in order to give the parents a chance to get some sleep and regain their energies and senses. Often knowing that they can take the baby to a relative or to hospital, can be a useful prop to the parents in coping with difficult situations and is seldom an offer that is abused. The problem of the crying baby is one where advice galore is offered but in the end it is the parents who have to find their own solution in managing the situation.

Toddlers and young children can likewise be poor sleepers and often these are the overactive children as well. The same considerations as previously mentioned apply. While the young mother has been rightfully concerned about her crying baby and disinclined to let it cry, for the toddler a firm approach is required. A sensible bedtime routine is required and once the child is settled in bed it should be made clear that it is bedtime and time to sleep. The parents should not rush back to every whim and disturbance and if they do go back it should be with indifference so that the child will not gain attention for his efforts. For the impossible child, sedation on a short term basis

Exclusion of organic causes

Chloral hydrate

Hospital admission as respite for parents

Toddlers who do not sleep

Bedtime routine

Sedation

with chloral hydrate or Vallergan forte in a pre-medication dose may be used. This may help the child get back to a normal sleep pattern. Many doctors are opposed on principle to giving night sedation for such children but due consideration has to be given to the parents if they are going to remain in a fit state to be responsible for their child. Sometimes it is the parents who need treatment. While it is said that the child will come to no harm without sleep, many such children are often irritable in the day-time and lack concentration. It is certainly true that the child's ability to endure sleeplessness is far greater than that of their parents. Many children come to their parents bed and contro-versy has existed over this for generations. If the parents do not mind and the family sleep satisfactorily, there seems little harm in it. The child as he gets older will inevitably prefer his own bed in any case. If the parents do mind their child coming to bed with them, then they must be consistent in their means of discour-aging him.

Risk of non-accidental injury

Much of the doctor's role in these problems is to be prepared to listen and sympathize. He must have a sense of when the situation is leading to breaking point (even in an apparently good home) and also to be very aware that many such instances can be either part of or lead to rejection of the child and to non-accidental injury.

The child who does not eat

Clinical assessment

Charting height and weight

This problem is frequently brought by the over-anxious parent. However, the doctor must never reject the problem out of hand since too rapid an assumption that the problem is entirely one of maternal anxiety, can lead to horrendous blunders. A clinical assessment of the child's overall progress and health is import-ant. It is very important to chart the child's height and weight on the percentile chart and in this respect if the child is falling significantly off his percentile growth, there is good reason to justify further investigation.

The majority of children are entirely normal on physical examination and are growing consistently along their expected centile. It is important to explain this to the parents in order to demonstrate the normality of their child's growth and in addition, to explain the fact that children tend to eat less avidly and more erratically between the age of about 2 years until the prepubertal growth spurt. Many young toddlers use food refusal as a weapon to gain the attention of their parents. As with temper tantrums, if ignored the problem becomes less. It is

Reassurance of parents

important to maintain the reassurance of the parents and in this respect extensive investigation is contraindicated since this tends to only heighten their anxiety about the possibility of organic disease. Most of these children eat what they like and not what their parents think they should eat. A record of all food eaten over a period is generally reassuring.

School problems

Most children do not like school at some stage. The majority endure this phase and emerge better for having coped successfully. Many children seem to have untold absences from school to the extent that schools these days are prepared to accept a certain degree of absence without question. Parental attitudes are very important and with certain trends against authority perhaps this is not surprising. Children from such homes who have frequent absences from school are usually those who tend to make the most of minor ailments.

Parental attitudes

Overt school refusal

Other children present with more overt school refusal causing great concern to their parents. Enquiries to the school (with parental consent) are important and often a visit by the health visitor or social worker may provide useful information as to the child's refusal to attend. In some instances the child may have a valid point in that there may be an undesirable teacher or there may be extreme unchecked bullying. It is important to know if the child is educationally suited to the school and if this is in question an educational psychologist's assessment may prove very useful.

Assessment of an educational psychologist

Child guidance clinic

Most difficulties are temporary but for the child in whom the problem seems complex and intractible, the help of the local child guidance clinic is probably the next best move. Undue delay in resolving such difficulties should be avoided, not only because the child's unhappiness may be profound, but because valuable educational time is being lost and never regained.

10 Developmental assessment and the handicapped child

Neonatal developmental assessment – Newborn reflexes and reactions – Special senses – General objectives in the assessment of the handicapped – Useful information

For far too long relatively little interest was shown in the handicapped child. Most paediatricians were too occupied in dealing with the acute illnesses of childhood but as the workload for this has diminished, interest in the handicapped child has grown. Regrettably the potential of reducing handicap by updating obstetric and perinatal care has not been fully realized. For those children born with handicaps it is important that the handicap is recognized early and its full nature assessed to identify the problems and plan a future to enhance the child's best potentials.

Early recognition and assessment

In order to recognize the abnormal it is important to be familiar with the normal. For this reason, in the care of infants and young children it is not only important to observe their growth and treat their illnesses, but also to note their developmental milestones. There is a fair range of variance in normal achievement and some children have a staircase-like type of development and an overall view of their development is necessary to gauge their progress. Some children will regress in their development as a consequence of illness, particularly if they are admitted to hospital, but they will quickly regain their milestones on recovery.

Referral for investigation and assessment

Once a child is spotted as having developmental delay, he should be referred for full investigation and assessment. There may well be a remedy for the developmental delay as in the case of congenital hypothyroidism. Where parents are worried about

115

their child's development, this is a justification for full assessment.

Development is a continuous process from conception to maturity and the sequence is the same in all children with concurrent sequences in different developmental fields. Development is clearly correlated with the development of the central nervous system and hence developmental milestones cannot precede neurological maturity and development is always in a cephalocaudal direction, hence head control precedes walking. It should be emphasized that developmental examinations are not tests of intelligence but, nevertheless, there is a fairly close association between the developmental quotient and subsequent intelligence. The following information can be reasonably obtained from developmental assessment in infancy.

(1) The comparison of the infant's development for his chronological age with the average of others of his age indicates his rate of development and gives an idea of his developmental potential. From this it is possible to diagnose moderate or severe mental subnormality.

(2) The diagnosis of significant neurological defects in infancy. This includes the diagnosis of cerebral palsy and the assessment of muscle tone.

(3) The detection of severe deafness and visual defects.

(4) The diagnosis of treatable conditions such as congenital hypothyroidism, phenylketonuria and congenital dislocation of the hips.

(5) As a result of this information it may be possible to achieve a diagnosis of the condition and realize the areas of handicap, hence affording guidance for therapy. Since some conditions are genetically determined it offers the opportunity of genetic counselling where it is equally important to be able to reassure parents that there are no significant genetic risks to a future pregnancy.

It should be equally realized that there are significant limitations to developmental assessment. Accurate predictions of future intelligence and achievements cannot be made especially since environmental factors will have much influence. It cannot be guaranteed that following assessment the child's ability will not subsequently deteriorate. Neurological signs detected in infancy, unless gross, may or may not disappear and one cannot

(margin notes)
Development and neurological maturity

Information to be gleaned for assessment

Limitations of assessment

predict whether later they may manifest as problems in co-ordination and special appreciation. The mildest cases of cerebral palsy or mental backwardness cannot always be diagnosed and likewise mild visual and hearing defects cannot always be detected early. Some factors cannot easily be scored such as alertness, general responsiveness and concentration, yet may be more relevant to future development and achievement than easily definable milestones.

The objective of developmental assessment is to determine that the child's development is normal for his age and whether he has any mental, physical, neurological or sensory handicaps that might benefit from appropriate treatment.

Scales of assessment
Several scales of assessment have been devised and among those commonly used are the Denver and Griffiths scales. These should not be confused with those used for intelligence testing.

Neonatal developmental assessment

Birth weight and gestational age
Initial assessment begins at birth and while most babies are born at term, some are pre-term. Birth weight is not a precise indicator of gestational age since some babies of low birth weight are small for gestational age. There is often a significant discrepancy between gestational age, calculated by dates from the last menstrual period and the actual gestational age but with

Ultrasound
the increasing use of ultrasound antenatally the estimation is much more precise. For babies of doubtful gestational age assessment using neurological and physical findings, such as those

Dubowitz scoring
scored on the Dubowitz scoring, can be quite useful in obtaining some idea as to whether the baby is pre-term or small for gestational age.

The early examination
The early newborn examination is important since the presence or absence of neurological signs at certain stages of development is often relevant to subsequent development. Ideally the baby should be examined about 2 hours after the last feed. Among the features to be observed are the following.

Chromosomal abnormalities
(1) The general appearance of the baby. The features of Down's syndrome are usually plainly apparent as are those of other chromosomal abnormalities.

Size of head
(2) The size of the head. Most full-term babies have a head circumference of about 35 cms. A grossly small head below the 3rd centile would indicate microcephaly,

117

whereas above the 97th centile could indicate raised intracranial pressure as caused by hydrocephaly.

(3) The general awareness of the baby; if he is unduly irritable or unresponsive. The nature of the cry may be significant.

(4) Posture. The normal full-term baby lying supine tends to keep his limbs flexed while a hypotonic baby lies in the 'surrender' position.

(5) Spontaneous movements may be abnormal – either jerky or obviously consistent with fitting. Alternatively there may be a poverty of movement.

(6) Muscle tone – this is difficult to define and is variable. Palpable consistency of the muscles and the range of limb movement gives some guide in this assessment. Some conclusion can usually be reached as to whether the baby has a normal muscle tone or is hypotonic.

Newborn reflexes and reactions

The rooting reflex

This is present in all full-term babies. When the baby's cheek touches the mother's breast he will root for the nipple. Likewise, when the examiner's finger touches the corner of the mouth the bottom lip is lowered and the tongue protruded to the point of stimulation and responses can be obtained in all four quadrants.

Not elicited in hungry baby
The reflex is not elicited when the baby is hungry.

Sucking and swallowing reflex
The sucking and swallowing reflexes are present in all but the smallest of pre-term babies. It is best tested by using a clean finger or teat. The absence of the sucking reflex either indicates significant neurologial impairment or the effects of sedation.

The Moro reflex

This is elicited by placing the baby supine and then lifting the head and neck about one inch above the mattress. On releasing support the reflex will be elicited.

The features of the reflex are abduction and extension of the arms with the hands open. This is followed by adduction of the arms as in an embrace. The baby inevitably cries and there is extension of the neck, trunk and legs. The Moro reflex is not to be confused with the startle response when the elbow remains flexed and the fist closed. The Moro reflex is a vestibular response and disappears at 3–4 months of age.

Significance   The significant variations in this reflex are that:

(1) The reflex is decreased in hypotonia and hypertonia,

(2) Decreased in cerebral damage and with sedation,

(3) It is asymmetrical due to hemiplegia or due to trauma to a limb,

(4) Increased in cerebral irritability.

The grasp reflex

Importance of head orientation

This is elicited by introducing a finger from the ulnar side of the palm of the hand and when the skin is stimulated the baby's fingers will grip the examiner's finger or object firmly. It is important that during the examination the baby's head should be in the midline otherwise the grasp will be stronger on the side to which the occiput is directed. Likewise the dorsum of the hand should not be touched as this induces an opposing reflex and the hand opens. The power of a baby's grasp is quite remarkable and in the full-term baby the grasping strength can be up to 2.2 kg. A similar reflex can be elicited by stroking the soles of the feet producing a grasp reflex of the toes. The palmar grasp reflex is maximal at term and diminishes at 2 months and has virtually disappeared by 3 months.

Significant features are:

(1) The symmetry and strength of the reflex are important. An exceptionally strong reflex can be found in cerebral palsy and kernicterus. It may be asymmetrical in hemiplegia.

(2) Persistence after 3 months may indicate spastic cerebral palsy.

Tonic neck reflexes

The asymmetrical tonic neck reflex is seen in young babies in the first 2 months of life. When the baby is supine and not crying he may lie with his head turned to one side with the arm extended on the same side. The contralateral knee is often flexed.

Significance   This reflex usually disappears at the age of 2–3 months but in severe cerebral palsy the reflex persists and may be

119

increased. The reflex is important in maintaining posture in the neonate and when persisting in the spastic child it presents problems in their bringing their hands to the midline or putting their hands to their mouth. It also impairs hand/eye co-ordination and prevents them from holding their head in the midline.

Eye reflexes

Blinking will occur on provocation by various stimuli including sound and bright light. The corneal reflex consists of blinking when the cornea is touched.

Doll's eye response

The doll's eye response is present in the first 10 days of life and is so named because there is delay in movement of the eyes when the head is turned.

Significance

The reflex usually disappears at 10 days when fixation develops but persists in abnormal babies. It is asymmetrical in abducens paralysis.

Lower limb reflexes

Crossed extension reflex

On flexing one leg the other leg flexes. The crossed extension reflex is elicited by holding one leg extended at the knee and stroking the sole of the foot on the same side. The other leg then flexes, adducts and then extends. This reflex disappears after the first month of life.

Placing and walking reflexes

The placing reflex is elicited by bringing the anterior aspects of the tibia against the edge of a table and the baby then lifts his leg as if to step onto the table. The walking reflex is obtained by holding the baby upright with his feet on the table so that the sole presses on the surface. This elicits a walking reflex but since the adductor muscles also contract, one leg tends to get caught behind the other. The walking reflex disappears at 5–6 months.

Significance

These reflexes are important in eliciting neurlological activity in babies with neural tube defects. Persistence of the reflex is seen in children with neurological damage.

The parachute reflex

This is a reflex that appears at 6–9 months and persists throughout life. It is elicited by holding the child in ventral suspension and suddenly throwing him forwards towards the couch. In doing this the arms extend as if to save him from falling.

Significance   In cerebral palsy the reflex is absent or incomplete owing to strong flexor tone. In the child with hemiplegia the response would be asymmetrical.

Tendon reflexes

These are relevant in the infant. The knee jerk elicited in the newborn if often associated with abduction of the opposite leg. The biceps, triceps and supinator jerks are easily elicited as is the ankle jerk.

Significance   Tendon reflexes are exaggerated in cerebral palsy and in disease of the pyramidal tracts the area over which the tendon jerks are elicited is greatly increased. The knee jerk can be elicited by tapping the dorsum of the foot or the triceps jerk by tapping the shoulder. Sustained ankle clonus often accompanies increased tendon reflexes. Isolated brisk reflexes are not themselves an indication of cerebral palsy and the diagnosis can only be made on assessment of the whole clinical picture.

Special senses

Vision

The newborn baby has a normal pupillary reaction to light. It is

Congenital catarract   always important to examine the eyes carefully for congenital cataract (which may be part of the rubella syndrome). By one

Focusing   month the baby should focus on his mother and by 3 months not only turn his eyes in the direction of an object but turn his head

Squints   as well. At this stage squints become apparent, being due to muscular incoordination and others due to intra-ocular lesions including retrolental fibroplasia. Many squints, however, are intermittent but should these persist beyond the age of 6 months an ophthalmological opinion should be sought.

Testing vision   Testing of vision in infancy is not always easy. The following steps should be followed.

(1) Birth–6 months: Observe the baby as to whether he focuses on his mother's face. His response to a bright light and whether he follows the light. Holding a toy brick to see if he will reach out for it and testing each eye independently.

121

(2) 6 months–2 years: Continued observation to see if the child is reacting as if he has normal vision. By 1 year the child should be able to pick up small objects with his finger and thumb and prior to this he should be following objects as they fall.

Rolling spheres test

Rolling spheres of varying sizes down to $\frac{1}{8}$ in across a piece of green baize is often used to test the vision of the infant. He is seated comfortably and the spheres are rolled across the baize in either direction 10 ft from where the child is sitting. The mother is also asked to cover each eye separately in order to test independent vision.

Stycar testing

(3) 2–4 years: The Stycar testing methods can be used with miniature matched toys placed 10 ft from the child. The examiner identifies his toy and the child is asked to match it.

(4) Children 5 years and older can be tested using the Stycar nine letter charts at 20 ft.

Snellen charts

(5) Children of 7 years and older can usually be tested with conventional Snellen charts.

Electro-retinogram

(6) In special instances an electroretinogram is indicated for retarded children with severe visual difficulties in order to try and identify whether their visual difficulties are ocular or cerebral.

Hearing

Language development

The testing of hearing is vitally important since language development cannot occur without normal hearing. The normal responses in infancy are:

Normal responses in infancy

1–2 months: when crying quietens to sound and vice versa.
3 months: turns head to sound made in the same plane.
6 months: turns to sound below the plane of the ear. Imitates sounds.
7 months: turns to sound above the ear.
12 months: turns on hearing own name.

Methods of testing

Mother's observation

(1) 0–6 months: observation of the baby's response to auditory stimuli. A mother's or a nurse's observations in this respect are very important.

Stycar and
Manchester
techniques

(2) 6–12 months: the use of simple materials and methods to test hearing such as the Stycar and Manchester techniques. Sit the baby comfortably on the mother's knee in a quiet room with minimal distraction. Materials used include the following:

> *The Stycar rattle*: shaking gently at 1 metre from the baby's head will produce a sound of 50 decibels and rotating 45 decibels.
>
> A cup and spoon: produces an easily recognizable sound above 40 decibels.
>
> Rustling toilet paper: 54 decibels.
>
> Kleenex tissue: 45 decibels.
>
> Crepe paper: used for higher frequencies 50–60 decibels.
>
> Stroking hair brush bristles: gives a higher frequency.
>
> Speech sounds: 'ah' and 'oo' 50 decibels, 'pe' and 'uss' 40 decibels.

For the child who seems profoundly deaf, ringing a bell or banging a drum may indicate some response to very loud noises. The use of the materials for testing is to see whether the baby can hear sounds within the range of the human speaking voice.

Free field
audiometer

(3) 1–3 years: the free field audiometer can be used which will give a greater idea of the child's specific hearing ability. Use of the human voice with certain words and asking a child to repeat them such as doll, dog, frog. Sets of pictures, asking the child to point to the object named e.g. peg/egg, moon/spoon, feet/sweet, pup/cup. This also affords some idea of verbal comprehension.

Conventional
audiometer

(4) 4 onwards: most children with normal intelligence can be tested using the conventional audiometer, asking them to stack up plastic cups each time an auditory response is elicited. When conducting the test it is very important to see that the child is not able to see the lever being pressed or any response from any of the dials because, on occasions, a clever deaf child has had an apparently normal audiogram because they have responded every time they have seen the operator depress the key. Should any deafness be elicited, impedence testing is useful to elicit any evidence of middle ear fluid.

Examination
of ears, nose
and throat

    Careful examination of the ears with the auroscope is always important as well as examination of the nose and throat.

123

Common causes of deafness

(1) Familial deafness,
(2) Rubella syndrome,
(3) Neonatal hyperbilirubinaemia
(4) Chronic otitis media,
(5) Severe perinatal anoxia,
(6) Alport's syndrome – congenital nephritis and deafness,
(7) Pendrict's syndrome – congenital goitre and deafness,
(8) Drugs – streptomycin, kanamycin and gentamicin in toxic dosages.

General objectives in the assessment of the handicapped

(1) To establish whether development is normal or abnormal.

(2) To establish a diagnosis and the nature of the handicap.

(3) To take appropriate measures:

    (i) Specific medical or surgical treatment,
    (ii) Appropriate education,
    (iii) To ensure the necessary support and aids are provided,
    (iv) Counselling and support for the family.

Regional Specialist Assessment Centres

Most paediatric departments provide for the handicapped child and so once the need for assessment is evident, referral to such a unit is justified so that the child and his family receive maximum support. There are Regional Specialist Assessment centres for the child with very complex problems or where parents rightly feel they would like a further opinion. Such units function on a multi-disciplinary basis which is essential in dealing with the complexities of the handicapped child. Members of these teams may include the following.

(1) A paediatrician to oversee the general problems of the child.

(2) A social worker.

(3) A physiotherapist.

(4) An occupational therapist.

(5) A speech therapist.

(6) Additional specialist opinions may be required from a

Local
facilities

paediatric neurologist, educational psychologist as well as from orthopaedic surgeons and ophthalmologists, some of whom take a special interest in the problems of the handicapped child.

On a local basis, the Community Medical Officers are trained in developmental assessment of children and are familiar with the local facilities that are available. Some districts have special assessment groups (for assessment and therapy) for infants while in others such facilities are either offered in nursery groups provided by special schools or by the local hospital. The schemes and facilities vary considerably from district to district and in dealing with such children it is important to be aware of what facilities are available.

A positive approach to the problems of the handicapped child not only enables the child to make the best of his potential abilities but support of the parents and family leads to a more rational acceptance of their child's problem and hopefully a better opportunity in life for their child.

Useful information

Organizations

MIND (National Association for Mental Health) 22, Harley Street, London, W1.

MENCAP (National Society for Mentally Handicapped Children) 117–123, Golden Lane, London EC17 0RT. Tel: 01-253 9433

The Downs Children's Association, Quinbourne Community Centre, Birmingham, B32 2TN. Tel: 021-427 1374

Spastic Society, 12, Park Crescent, London W1N 4EQ. Tel: 01-636 5021

Muscular Dystrophy Group of Great Britain, 35, Macauly Road, London, SW4 0QP. Tel: 01-720 8055

Disable Living Foundation, 346, Kensington High Street, London, W14 8NS. Tel: 01-602 2491

Association for Spina Bifida and Hydrocephalus, Tavistock House, North Tavistock Square, London, WC1. Tel: 01-388 1382

Invalid Childrens Aid Association, 126, Buckingham Palace Road, London, SW1 W9SB. Tel: 01-730 9891

National Deaf Childrens Society, 31, Gloucester Place, London W1H 4EA. Tel: 01-486 3251/2

Royal National Institute for the Deaf, 105, Gower Street, London WC1E 6AH. Tel: 01-387 8033

Royal National Institute for the Blind, 224–8, Great Portland Street, London W1N 6AA. Tel: 01-388 1266

11 Surgical conditions

Common surgical conditions – Abnormalities of the female external genitalia – The umbilicus – Hare lip, cleft palate and tongue tie – Swellings in the neck – Ear, nose and throat surgery – The eyes – Neurosurgical conditions – Orthopaedic problems

While it is well recognized that medical problems in children differ from adults, likewise paediatric surgery differs in that many operations are performed to enable the child to return to a normal growth and development as opposed to only reconstruction surgery in the mature adult. The old tradition that the newborn baby should have the minimal surgery required and, if possible, to defer action until the child is older, is now completely outmoded. In relation to age the technical aspects and the physiological and psychological responses vary and require full consideration in management. While there are an increasing number of paediatric surgeons, some have specialized in fields such as cardiac surgery, urology and neurosurgery, but at district hospital level most children's surgery is done by the general surgeon. It is fortunately not uncommon to find at least one member of such a team who takes a special interest in paediatric surgery.

Admission of young children to hospital can be upsetting and so most are admitted for the shortest period necessary. For some surgical procedures they are admitted as day cases provided the family conditions are good for them to return home.

Common surgical conditions

Inguinal hernia

This occurs in 1 in 50 boys and 1 in 400 girls by the age of 12 years. Most hernias are indirect with a peritoneal sac extruding from the internal inguinal ring down the very short inguinal canal to present at the external inguinal ring at the groin or extend further into the scrotum.

Clinical findings

Intermittent

A symptomless swelling in the groin is the most common present-ation. It may extend into the scrotum. The swelling is often inter-mittent owing to the reducibility of the hernia. The older child often complains of discomfort and babies may seem in dis-comfort as well, crying noticeably less after surgical repair. If the swelling can be reduced with an audible or palpable gurgle there is little doubt about the diagnosis. If there is no gurgle this may be due to fluid or omentum in the sac. When fluid is absent

'Silk sign'

the 'silk sign' can be elicited by rubbing the finger across the spermatic cord and pressing it against the pubic bone, a typical rustling feeling is elicited when a hernial sac is present.

Differential diagnosis

This rests between a hernia or a hydrocele. The difference is that a hernia is a swelling which is inguinal or inguinal scrotal extending downwards, whereas a hydrocele is a scrotal swell-ing extending upwards. As a result of this, one can always palpate the cord above the hydrocele but not with a hernia.

Transillumin-ation

Transillumination of a hydrocele may be a useful additional sign but is not diagnostic.

Hernias in girls

In girls the ovary may enter the hernial sac and feels similar to a hydrocele of the canal of Nuck. Since 2–4% of inguinal hernias in females are associated with testicular feminization, a buccal smear or chromosome studies are indicated (specimens can be taken while the child is under anaesthetic).

Strangulated hernia

Testicular atrophy

This is a tense, tender irreducible swelling, most often occurring in the first year of life. About 10% are followed by testicular atrophy of some degree.

Management and treatment

Rapid
treatment
Spontaneous
resolution
under 6 weeks

Surgery

It is important that once a hernia is diagnosed, even though it is reducible, it should be operated on at the earliest convenient opportunity. In babies under the age of 6 weeks it may be reasonable to defer surgery as some will resolve spontaneously but beyond this age it is unknown for a hernia to disappear. Leaving a hernia exposes the baby to the risk of strangulation and encarceration with a significantly higher risk than for elective surgery. Some surgeons prefer to explore both sides at the time of operation since there is a significant risk of a hernia arising on the contralateral side. Current feeling tends to prefer leaving the other side since most parents seek early advice if there is any sign of a hernia developing.

A strangulated hernia requires immediate admission to hospital for reduction and then herniotomy. Usually gentle pressure will reduce the hernia but for others sedation is required along with elevation of the foot of the bed or suspension of the infant in gallows traction.

Trusses have no place in the treatment of hernias today except possibly to keep a hernia reduced while the child recovers from another condition.

Hydrocele

This is a collection of fluid in a persistent part of the processus vaginalis. It may or may not have communication with the abdomen but it is occasionally large enough to allow abdominal contents to enter, a 'communicating' hydrocele. Usually the infant has a small non-tense bilateral scrotal swelling which, under normal circumstances, resolves in the first year of life. Should there be a unilateral tense hydrocele, this is less likely to resolve but it is still reasonable to wait until the child is a year of age before considering surgery.

Clinical presentation

Hydrocele presents as a symptomless swelling in the scrotum which may extend up to the inguinal ring. The swelling will transilluminate but it should be remembered that a hernia may transilluminate as well. The swelling is along the line of the spermatic cord but above the testis and below the inguinal ring.
Surgery is only seriously considered for the large hydrocele

129

after the age of 1 year. It should be remembered that post-surgery a scrotal swelling may persist for some time and it is important to explain this to the parents.

Torsion of the testis

Immediate action

This is a condition where immediate recognition and action are vital if the testis is to be viable. Torsion occurs because in some the testis hangs on a mesorchium from the epididymis and hence is liable to rotate. In others the cord may undergo torsion above the testis. Torsion of the testis tends to be relatively more common in the incompletely descended testis although the majority occur in the normal. The anatomical anomaly tends to be bilateral and hence the need surgically to prophylactically fix the other side at the time of operation. Although torsion is common in the school age it can occur in infancy and even in the neonatal period.

Prophylactic surgery

Clinical findings

The presentation is usually sudden pain and swelling in one testis which may produce reflex vomiting. The testis is swollen and tender. Partial torsion, however, can give rise to less severe symptoms which can be confused with epididymo-orchitis.

In all cases immediate referral for surgical exploration is essential.

Epididymo-orchitis

Response to antibiotics

This presents as a firm tender swelling in the epididymis which may also involve the testis. It may be due to infection from the urinary tract or from haematogenous spread. It usually responds well to antibiotics but untreated may produce a discharging sinus. Staphylococcal orchitis tends to occur in the neonatal period and early infancy. A chronic infection may be tuberculous in origin. Mumps produces an acute orchitis and occasionally this can present before a parotid swelling.

TB
Mumps

Differential diagnosis

Surgical exploration

This is between torsion of the testis especially if this is partial. In the absence of definite evidence of infection it is important to refer these patients since they may require surgical exploration.

130

Varicocele

Wilmer's
tumour of
kidney

Oligospermia
in adult

This may be present in the adolescent but is rare in younger children where, if it does occur, it is reported as an association with a Wilmer's tumour of the kidney. In the uncomplicated situation it is associated with oligospermia in adult life and hence justifies treatment.

Undescended testes

There are three groups of conditions in relation to descent of the testes.

(1) The retractile testis which is a normal varient and requires no treatment at all.

(2) The incompletely descended testis.

(3) The ectopic testis.

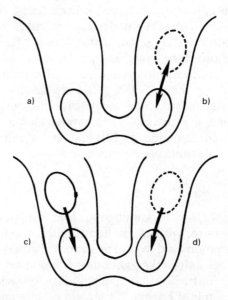

a) Normal testis
b) Retractile testis to superficial inguinal pouch
c) Superficial ectopic testis in front of the inguinal canal but will not manipulate into the scrotum
d) The inguinal emergent testis palpable in the inguinal canal but will not manipulate into the scrotum

Conditions relating to the descent of the testes

Figure 11.1

131

Problems in Paediatrics

Incidence

It was shown by Scorer and Farrington that 3.4% of all newborn
have incomplete descent of the testis and up to 30.3% of
premature babies. By 1 year there is an overall incidence of
0.27% and this figure correlates well with an incidence of
0.28% in school children. This implies that, apart from the
retractile testis, spontaneous descent is rare after the age of 1
year.

Pathology

Patent processus vaginalis
Histological abnormality

About 50% of incompletely descended testes will have a patent
processus vaginalis and a few will be associated with an
inguinal hernia. Electron microscopy has shown differences in
histology from the normal from early infancy and light microscopy changes are apparent after the age of 5 years. These
changes have been described as dysplasia which is essentially a
failure to mature. It has also been found that similar changes
are found in about a third of the contralateral testes. It has been
suggested that a lack of testosterone, probably secondary to a
lack of pituitary stimulus, may be a part of the condition.

Hormonal deficiency

Associated conditions

Certain conditions are associated with undescended testes
and these include the triad syndrome of abdominal wall
agenesis, obstructive uropathy and cryptocordism. Hypopituitism is associated with hypogonadism. Some chromosomal
abnormalities such as Klinefelter's syndrome are associated
with bilateral cryptocordism.

Examination

Warm, relaxed atmosphere

It is important to examine the child in a warm room and relaxed
atmosphere, with warm hands. All too many circumstances of
examination tend to lead to a rapid disappearance of the retractile testis before the examination has scarcely begun. The child
should firstly be examined standing to see if there is any associated inguinal hernia. He should be examined lying down with
his legs slightly abducted and then, placing the fingers of the one
hand medial to the anterior superior iliac spine, gentle pressure
is applied along the inguinal canal down to the external ring.
While the pressure is maintained the testis is palpated in the
scrotum with the other hand.

Chair test

The chair test is useful to elicit the retractile testis. The
child sits comfortably on a chair and is then asked to put his

132

hands round his knees and pull his knees hard on to his chest. This relaxes the cremasteric muscle and if the testis is retractile it will descend into the scrotum.

Management

Surgery

Children over 1 year in whom the testis is not descended (excluding the retractile testis) should be referred for a further opinion, either to a paediatrician or directly to an appropriate surgeon. Recommendations of the age for surgery have varied – most prefer to operate before school age but some defer action to the age of 8 or 9 years.

Fertility

Malignancy

In later life most of those with unilateral cryptocordism have normal fertility but of those with bilateral cryptocordism only 4% have normal fertility. Although the risk of malignancy in the undescended testes is 30 times greater than in the descended testes, the overall risk is remote.

Circumcision

It is accepted that circumcision is not routinely indicated and can, in fact, carry a small but significant mortality and morbidity. Some children are circumcized on religious grounds and it is

Religious grounds

important to see that they are medically fit prior to this being done. This includes checking that the baby is not significantly premature or jaundiced and that there is no family history of bleeding disorders and no evidence of hypospadias. Among the

Medical indications for circumcision

medical indications for circumcision are:

(1) Phimosis – it is important to realize that the foreskin is adherent to the glans at birth and usually separates at about the age of 1 year. In the child whose foreskin will not retract after the age of 2 years the foreskin is often long and urine collects in the distal sac giving rise to chronic inflammatory change and fibrosis leading to a phimosis.

(2) Paraphimosis occurs when the foreskin is long but has become adherent to the glans. It can be forcibly retracted but the contracted ring of the foreskin becomes irreducibly stuck over the rim of the glans.

(3) Recurrent balanitis – it is important to differentiate

Ammoniacal dermatitis

between infection within the subprepucial pocket and ammoniacal dermatitis giving external redness to the foreskin. In the latter situation circumcision is absolutely contraindicated since the foreskin is protecting the glans from ammoniacal burning and preventing scarring of the urethral meatus leading to a meatal stricture.

Stretching the foreskin and probing to separate adhesions are only of marginal benefit and in most instances it is better to directly perform a circumcision.

Micropenis

This is a rare condition. More commonly this is erroneously diagnosed when a normal penis is buried in a large pad of supra-pubic fat, in the obese child, known as the 'toad-in-the-hole' penis. A small diameter of the penile shaft is more significant in terms of failure of development than length.

Hypospadias

This is a common anomaly occurring in 1 in 300 males and is of varying severity. In extreme forms intersex problems should be considered.

Urethral deficiency
    Hypospadias is a condition in which the anterior urethra is deficient to a varying degree so that the urethral meatus can be found anywhere from the usual site to the perineum. The following types can be distinguished.

(1) Glandular hypospadias – is when the glandular urethra is missing, giving rise to a groove on the under-surface of the glans. It may give rise to problems due to a ventral diversion of the urinary stream. There is no chordii and so the penis erects normally. The condition is usually associated with a hooded foreskin. If there is any evidence of meatal stricture, it is important to note that there are no significant back-pressure changes. Depending on the severity, only minor surgical correction of this condition is required.

Normal penile erection

Meatal stricture

(2) Penile hypospadias – is when the urethral opening is displaced further back than the coronal sulcus. It is always accompanied by some degree of chordii. This condition certainly requires surgery which is a two stage procedure, firstly the release of the chordii followed later by reconstruction of the urethra.

Two stage surgery

(3) Perineal hypospadias – is when the urethra opens onto the perineum and the scrotum is cleft by a persistent urogenital groove. In some instances these cases appear as an intersex and will require investigation accordingly.

Investigation for intersex

Multistage
surgery
    The condition obviously requires surgical correction and this is usually a multistage procedure.

Renal
anomalies
    About 5% of children with hypospadias have associated renal anomalies. Renal ultrasound is the best method of investigating this at present.

Rectal prolapse

This is more often seen in children with chronic diarrhoea and it
Cystic fibrosis is most important to realize its association with cystic fibrosis.
Treatment   The prolapse is kept reduced by strapping the buttocks. Avoidance of straining at stool is important and also ensuring that the child does not squat on defaecation. Most resolve within a year but some require injection with sclerosing agents.

Rectal bleeding

Neonates occasionally strain at stool and produce a little blood but this usually harmless and ceases spontaneously. In the ill neonate it is obviously important to consider such conditions as necrotizing enterocolitis and haemorrhagic disease of the newborn.

Anal abrasions

A small fissure *in ano* can be produced by constipation giving rise to the stool being streaked with fresh blood. If the fissure is
Anaesthetic painful a local anaesthetic ointment relieves the symptoms and
ointment usually these heal without problem. If the constipation is long-
Stool standing stool softening agents (such as Duphalac or Dioctyl-
softeners Medo) and modification of diet may be required.

Rectal polyps

In children these are mainly haematomatous. They are benign and develop in the mucosal layer. Most are palpable on rectal examination and some develop a false pedicle by traction on the mucosa. They may be single or multiple and give rise to dark red blood mixed with mucus.

Juvenile polyposis coli

This is a benign condition which can occur in the first decade of life. It is familial. The blood loss, however, may be severe enough to justify colectomy but otherwise the condition is treated expectantly.

Familial adenomatous polyposis coli

Pre-malignant

This rarely presents in the first decade of life. It is inherited as an autosomal dominant trait with a high degree of penetrance. As it is known to be a pre-malignant condition elective colectomy and iliorectal anastomosis are indicated.

Peutz–Zeaghar syndrome

This is a condition associated with polyps in the small intestine. They may give rise to intussusception. The condition is associated with brown pigmented spots in the circum oral area.

Meckel's diverticulum

Heavy rectal bleeding

Laparotomy

This may give rise to considerable rectal bleeding due to ulceration of ectopic mucosa within the diverticulum. Investigations to identify this are not entirely reliable, hence laparotomy is indicated.

Abnormalities of the female external genitalia

Vaginal skin tag

In neonates it is not uncommon to find a skin tag at the posterior forchette. It does not require any treatment.

Adherent labia

This is usually a midline fusion of the labia minora. They can usually be gently separated with a probe, after which it is important for the mother to apply a little Vaseline after washing the baby in order to prevent further fusion.

Microcolpus

This is due to obstruction of the genital tract. There are two forms:

(1) Imperforate hymen
(2) Vaginal atresia

Owing to obstruction, the uterus and sometimes also the fallopian tubes, are distended with secretions. Mucocolpus may present as abdominal swelling at birth and the pressure of the distended uterus may compress the large bowel to produce constipation.

Haematocolpus

Presents at menarche

The presents at the menarche with abdominal pain, absence of menstrual flow and occasionally retention of urine. On palpation there is a large abdominal mass due to the distended uterus.

Vaginal atresia

The condition is treated by a cruciate incision of the hymen. Vaginal atresia is much rarer and requires major surgical reconstruction.

The umbilicus

Umbilical granuloma

The umbilical cord usually separates within the first 5–7 days of life. Occasionally an umbilical granuloma will appear in the stump as a red, moist globular swelling consisting of granulomatous tissue.

Treatment

Frequent swabbing with spirit is usually effective in treating this condition. For the more persistent lesion, cautery of the granuloma with a silver nitrate stick can be used and if the granuloma is pedunculated it can be ligated at the base with a silk suture.

Patent vitaline duct

Occasionally the embryonic vitaline duct may remain patent and this also gives rise to a red moist swelling at the umbilicus. Within the swelling may be peritoneum or even bowel. If this is thought to be the case, surgical exploration is required.

Single umbilical artery

This has a frequent association with congenital defects including urinary tract anomalies which occur in 1% of those with a single vessel. Renal ultrasound at present is probably the best method of investigating the renal tract.

137

Umbilical hernia

Spontaneous resolution

True umbilical hernias protrude directly through the thick-walled ring of the abdominal wall at the umbilicus. The hernial sac is usually spherical in shape and is easily reduced and encarceration is very rare. It results from failure of closure of the prenatal umbilical ring but the process of closure can occur after birth so that the majority of hernias resolve spontaneously by the age of 1 year.

No treatment is necessary since all invariably resolve.

Associated conditions

Other medical conditions associated with umbilical hernia should be borne in mind and these include hypothyroidism, gargoylism and in the neonate, ascites and abdominal swelling due to an enlarged viscus. The majority of hernias otherwise appear in normal healthy children and seem more prevalent among the West Indians than the Caucasian.

Para-umbilicial hernia

Surgical repair

This is a protrusion through a transverse elliptical slit, usually just above the umbilical ring, but occasionally below. The typical swelling is conical and protrudes downwards. While the very small hernia may resolve spontaneously, most do not. Encarceration is rare and so it is reasonable to consider surgical repair at about the age of 4 years.

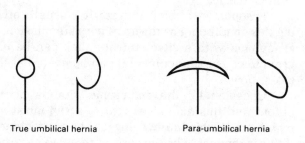

True umbilical hernia   Para-umbilical hernia

Figure 11.2

Appearance of umbilical herniae

Exomphalus

Amniotic sac

This is a larger herniation at the umbilicus where a sac is formed by amnion and not by skin. There are two types:

138

Surgical conditions

    (1) Those that herniate into the cord through a narrow base but may contain most of the mid gut and

    (2) Those with a wide base which may contain viscera as well as gut.

Associated anomalies

It should be noted that there is a high incidence of anomalies associated with exomphalus, including a significant incidence of cardiac anomalies.

Management

Firstly careful delivery of the baby is important in order to avoid rupturing the omphocele.

Protective covering

A sterile plastic bag such as a urine collecting bag can be trimmed to form a non-adherent cover with dressings used to build up round the edge in order to avoid the ompholocele hanging and constricting the blood supply. Saline packs and gauze are best avoided as they have the disadvantage of chilling

Surgery

the baby unduly. The baby should then be transferred to a paediatric surgeon and the plan of action will depend on the size of the exomphalus, smaller defects being primarily closed at an early stage whereas this may not be possible in the larger defects until the child is 18 months to 2 years of age.

Hare-lip, cleft palate and tongue tie

Hare lip and cleft palate

This is a relatively uncommon condition with an incidence of 1 in 1000 live births. Owing to the skills of plastic surgery the outcome is usually very satisfactory.

It is usual to repair the hare-lip at about the age of 3 months and to repair the palate at 1 year of age. While most lesions are obvious, careful examination of the palate is most important in order to detect a cleft of the soft palate.

Management

Problems that arise are not usually surgically related and include:

Feeding problems

    (1) Feeding – this is difficult in many babies with a cleft palate although some will breast feed without problem and otherwise will feed from a bottle with a teat with an enlarged hole. A flanged teat is of help and permits normal sucking action but it does tend to ulcerate the edges of the cleft, increasing the risk of infection and

139

Spoon feeding

making later surgery more difficult. Spoon feeding is therefore recommended and most mothers can easily be taught the technique of spooning milk into the baby's cheek without too much air or milk to induce choking.

Risk of infection

(2) These children are vulnerable to upper respiratory tract infections and middle ear infection. Where possible it is best to keep them away from others with upper respiratory tract infection and perhaps to prescribe antibiotics more readily than one would do otherwise. It is important to keep the nasal airway clear since these babies are unable to sneeze effectively.

Orthodontic supervision

(3) Orthodontic supervision is important since many clefts will involve the alveolus as well as the palate and lip.

Speech therapy and hearing tests

(4) A speech therapist's supervision is likewise important, particularly in the less straightforward cases. Speech therapists are usually very good on advising in feeding techniques. Regular hearing tests should be performed especially when language development is in question.

Tongue-tie

Overdiagnosis

This is a ridiculously over-diagnosed condition in welfare clinics. In infancy the anterior third of the tongue is short, giving a false impression of tongue-tie. There are, however, a few children where the frenulum extends to the tip of the tongue which is tethered. Although it does not cause significant feeding or speech difficulties, it can cause trivial difficulties later if the frenulum does not stretch, such as being unable to lick an ice-cream etc.

Surgery

In these children it is reasonable to divide the frenulum under general anaesthesia since the lingular artery and the submandibular ducts are all too easy to accidentally sever. It is advisable to wait until the infant is at least 9 months of age before considering action.

Ranula

This is a cystic swelling under the tongue. It requires marsupialization, otherwise recurrence is common.

Swellings in the neck

Branchial cyst

This develops under the upper third of the sternomastoid and extends outwards as it enlarges. It is a slow-growing, soft, cystic

Embryological
remnant

swelling and requires surgical excision. Embryologically it is a remnant of the second branchial cleft.

Arising from the same embryonic remnant a branchial sinus can arise and presents as a pinhead-sized pit on the anterior border of the lower third of the sternomastoid muscle. It may become infected and discharge on the neck and surgical exploration and excision is indicated.

Cervical lymph nodes

These are commonplace in association with upper respiratory tract infections and in conditions of the skull. Most of the lymph nodes are small, mobile and discreet and usually gradually disappear, although often not for several months.

Lymphomas

Rarely lymphomas occur in childhood but should cervical lymph nodes be rubber in consistency, persistent and without any obvious underlying infective cause, then a biopsy should be considered.

Sternomastoid tumours

Spontaneous
resolution

These probably arise from trauma of the sternomastoid muscle at birth. It is usually felt as a swelling in the lower third of the muscle. Most resolve spontaneously in the first 2 months of life but some will lead to shortening of the muscle and to torticollis.

Surgery

Treatment is teaching the mother to stretch the muscle and daily exercises in early infancy and later, if torticollis still develops, surgical division of the sternomastoid muscle is required.

Midline swellings

Thyroglossal cyst

This is found either on or just below the hyoid bone. It is firm and pea-sized and surgical removal is indicated. There is a tendency to recurrence if a remnant is left.

Thyroid gland

Hyper- and hypothyroid conditions are mostly treated medically but uncontrolled thyrotoxicosis is an indication for subtotal thyroidectomy.

Ear, nose and throat surgery (see Chapter 2)

One of the problems of early childhood is recurrent respiratory tract infections. Some parents often press for something to be done but in the ordinary situation this is not necessary. In the past, routine tonsillo-adenoidectomy was inept but having exposed the not insignificant dangers we are perhaps now a little too reluctant to consider the merits of removing either the tonsils or the adenoids.

Tonsils

Indications for tonsillectomy are:

Indications for
tonsillectomy

(1) Genuine recurrent tonsillitis. This is at least four proven infections a year. Probably there are many children who have undue time off school with tonsillar infection quite unnecessarily because of a reluctance to remove the tonsils.

(2) Peritonsillar abscess and tuberculous infection of the tonsils are rare in this country but do indicate tonsillectomy when the initial infection is cured.

(3) Enormous tonsils which threaten to produce airway obstruction. This is an uncommon indication for tonsillectomy but an important one. Many children otherwise

Large tonsils

have large tonsils and it should be remembered that lymphoid tissue grows until the child is 7 years of age and then slowly regresses.

Adenoids

There are probably stronger indications to remove the adenoids than the tonsils. Indications for adenoidectomy are as follows:

Indications for
adenoid-
ectomy

(1) The child with either recurrent middle ear infection or secretory otitis media with deafness, associated with adenoidal hypertrophy.

(2) The chronic nasal breather with obvious adenoidal facies who snores at night. Many of these children fail to thrive because of difficulty in eating owing to the blocked nasal airway.

Nasal polyps

These are uncommon but do occasionally cause nasal obstruction and require removal. There is a significant association with cystic fibrosis.

Myringotomy and grommets

This is indicated in cases of secretory otitis media associated with deafness. There is no clear evidence of the best way to treat this condition. Some evidence favours conservative measures as being as effective.

Eyes (See Problems in Ophthalmology – Glasspool)

Strabismus

Squints are important to refer to the ophthalmologist as soon as possible since, in order to develop normal stereo-optic vision, proper alignment of the visual axes is essential. Many babies have intermittent squinting in the early months of life but a
Persistent squint
persistent squint after the age of 6 months requires further investigation.

Blocked tear ducts

Blocked tear ducts result from chronic decrocystitis. Regular ocular toilet and, if necessary, antibiotics are required. In
Massage
addition it is important to massage the inner canthus of the eye with the little finger as this helps dislodge debris from the naso-lachrymal duct and maintain patency. Those cases that do not resolve on conservative treatment may require probing.

Retrolental fibroplasia

P_a,O_2 levels
Although monitoring of arterial P_a,O_2 levels in premature babies is more sophisticated and accurate than previously, cases of retrolental fibroplasia still occur. Preterm babies of 30 weeks gestation and less who have required oxygen therapy should be
Laser coagulation
checked for this condition regularly. Laser coagulation may afford a technique of preventing advance of this disease and subsequent blindness.

Neurosurgical conditions

Hydrocephalus

Increased CSF volume
This is a condition in which the volume of CSF proportion to the other cranial contents is greater than normal, giving rise to

enlargement of the ventricular system internally and possibly also enlargement of the subarachnoid space externally. The condition can occur at any age and it may be static or can progress at any time.

Causes

Hydrocephalus arises from impaired CSF circulation and may be caused by congenital malformation of the brain, neoplasm, bacterial meningitis and cranial trauma. Since CSF production from the choroid plexi continues to be produced irrespective of any blockage, it gives rise to ventricular enlargement and distension as far down as the site of obstruction.

Clinical signs

In infants the rate of growth of the skull will increase in response to rising intracranial pressure. The fontanelles will enlarge and bulge and the sutures will widen. It is always important, therefore, to regularly measure and chart the infants' skull circumference and note any sudden change in growth rate. As the intracranial pressure increases the infant

'Setting sun' eyes and globular head

develops the 'setting sun' appearance of the eyes and a globular shaped head with a percussion note likened to percussing a ripe water melon. Drowsiness, irritability, regression in motor milestones and vomiting will occur.

Older children

In older children where the sutures may have fused, the symptoms of raised intracranial pressure develop earlier with irritability and vomiting, limb tremor, ataxia and 6th cranial nerve palsy.

Investigations

Skull X-ray

(1) Skull X-ray is useful to indicate widening of the sutures and on occasions will show cranial calcification.

CAT scan

(2) Computerized axial tomography (CAT scan) is probably the current means of establishing a diagnosis. Prior to this air encephalography was required.

Treatment

Shunt operation

The majority of cases of hydrocephalus with rising intracranial pressure are treated with a shunt operation. Less commonly, according to circumstance, choroid plexotomy, ventriculo-cisternotomy and medical treatment with isosorbide are also used.

The shunts are either ventriculo-atrial or more commonly ventriculo-peritoneal. These shunts are plastic tubes which are inserted into the dilated ventricles and attached to a pressure release valve. The tubing is tracked down under the skin to drain into the peritoneum or into the jugular vein and down into the right atrium.

Problems related to treatment with a shunt are:

Problems with shunts

Low intracranial pressure

Blockage

(1) The shunt may be too effective at first and produce low intracranial pressure. This is unwanted since it is liable to give rise to a subdural haematoma owing to traction on the cortical veins.

(2) Blockage or disconnection of the tube giving rise to further raised intracranial pressure.

Infection

(3) Infection of the ventriculo-atrial shunt can give rise later to bacteraemia, chronic ill health, anaemia and spleno-megaly.

Aspiration

The valves can be pumped to check their patency. It is very important not to aspirate CSF with a syringe needle through the tubing as it gives rise to a permanent leak. Some shunts have an attached reservoir and if the location of this is known aspiration in emergency situations is acceptable.

Shunt failure

If there is any serious doubt about the system working, the neurosurgical unit who performed the operation should be contacted and, failing that, the nearest paediatric unit.

Subdural haematoma/effusion

Trauma

High mortality in young adults

This can occur at any age resulting from a trauma to the head. Except in infancy and the elderly it usually forms part of a severe complex cranial injury and hence there is a high mortality in young adults. In infancy subdural haematomas arise either from accidental or non-accidental trauma and non-blood-stained effusions can be a complication of bacterial meningitis.

Clinical presentation is as follows:

(1) Vomiting is a frequent initial symptom.

(2) Fits, which may present in the baby as apnoeic attacks.

145

(3) Irritability and failure to thrive.

(4) Signs of raised intracranial pressure.

(5) Anaemia.

Management

Immediate hospital admission
Suspicion of a subdural collection in a child requires immediate admission to a paediatric unit who, in turn, would seek neuro-surgical assistance. Acute effusions often resolve after aspiration but some may become chronic and require a shunt operation (subdural pleural shunt). While most children survive

Prognosis
to be normal, it is noted that up to 10% die and that about 20% are later mentally subnormal.

Brain tumours

Intracranial tumours in children are rare but important to recognize. Among the neoplastic disease in children, apart from

Incidence
the leukaemias, they are the most common. In the United Kingdom between 180–200 children are diagnosed annually as having intracranial tumours. Most neoplasms in children tend to arise in the posterior fossa but not exclusively.

Table 11.1 Common symptoms on presentation of intracranial tumours (analysis of 303 cases in children under 13)

Vomiting	186
Headache	148
Unsteady limbs or gait	128
Impaired consciousness	111
Strabismus	58
Limb weakness	36
Seizures	34
Impaired vision	12
Enlarged head	11
Dysarthria	4
Dysphagia	3

From 'Paediatric Neurosurgery'.

Prognosis
The prognosis depends on the nature and site of the neoplasm as well as the duration of symptoms. Prompt referral is therefore imperative. The clinical signs will depend on the site

Mydriatics contra-indicated
of the lesion. Examination of the fundi in children is not easy but it should be remembered that *mydriatics are absolutely contra-indicated if raised intracranial pressure is suspected.*

146

Surgical conditions

Spinal dysraphism

Congenital structural malformations involve the central nervous system more than any other part of the body. With regard to spinal abnormalities, meningomyelocele is the most common but there are other lesions that deserve attention. These include:

Meningo-
myelocele

> dermal sinus,
> lipoma and,
> diastematomyelia.

Retained

Extension of
spinal cord

In the embryo the lower part of the spinal cord degenerates to leave a thin thread of filium terminale. This degeneratory process does not always occur and in this case there is an extension of the spinal cord which is attached to the posterior dura. Associated with this may be a number of fibrous bands running from skin or bone to dura and hence the elongated cord. Occasionally there is a mesodermal growth in the form of a lipoma which has both subcutaneous and cord attachments. Skin ectoderma may remain attached to the neuroectoderma to form a dermoid cyst either within or adjacent to the cord or there may be a connection to the epidermis through a dermal sinus. In other cases there may be splitting of the motor cord responsible for duplication of the spinal column, usually in the form of a bony spur dividing the spinal cord into two halves. This is called diastematomyelia which is associated with an elongated and tethered cord.

Diastemat-
omyelia

Importance of
investigation

These defects can give rise to neurological signs in the lower limbs as well as affecting sphincter control. Investigation of children in respect of such lesions is important as appropriate surgery to release the cord may save advance of neurological signs.

Orthopaedic problems

This is an extensive subject and many conditions are uncommon but among the more frequent encountered conditions are the following.

Congenital dislocation of the hips

Early
diagnosis

This is one of the most important conditions to diagnose in early infancy. Correct diagnosis at or soon after birth carries a good prognosis with simple measures but late diagnosis when the

147

child is walking involves open surgery to the hip and often a less than satisfactory result. The incidence of congenital dislocation varies between 4–11 per 1000 live births and 8–20 per 1000 live births for dislocatable hips.

Predisposing factors

The cause of congenital dislocation of the hips is unknown but among the well recognized predisposing factors are:

(1) Females are more commonly affected than males with a 3–5 times greater incidence.

(2) Breech presentation, particularly females, are commonly more affected.

(3) In families where the condition has already occurred there is a 5% incidence.

(4) In monozygotic twins, if one is affected, there is a 40% chance of the other also being affected.

(5) Families of Mediterranean ancestery have a high incidence.

(6) Other orthopaedic anomalies including talipes and arthrogryphosis have a known association.

(7) Undue muscle laxness.

Importance of examination in first year

In most maternity units the babies are routinely examined by the paediatric staff. Although the baby may be declared 'normal' after examination it should be remembered that it is not impossible to miss a congenital hip dysplasia on initial examination and there may be some who subsequently genuinely dislocate within the first few months of life. *The hips therefore should not only be examined on every newborn examination but on every routine examination during the first year of life.*

Diagnosis

Essential signs

This is made on clinical examination, especially since the radiological appearances are not helpful until 3–4 months of age when the head of the femur begins to ossify. The essential signs to elicit are:

Lower limb contours

(1) Inspection of the lower limb contours with the infant supine. Asymmetrical skin folds may be normal but an additional fold suggests telescoping of the limb. With the limbs extended the perineum should not be visible and if it

148

is it would suggest bilateral subluxation (easy to miss as there is no normal for comparison).

Abduction of thighs

(2) The thighs are flexed and abducted fully and should abduct to about 90°. An abduction of less than 60–70° indicates an abnormality.

Stability of hip joint

(3) The stability of the hip joint should be evaluated to see if the femoral head is displacable from the acetabulum. With the infant supine the knees are flexed and the thighs are held in the palm of the hand with the 3rd finger laterally placed over the greater trochanter and the thumb placed medially just below the inguinal groove. With the thighs in mid abduction lateral pressure can then be applied with the fingers and medial pressure applied with the thumb. In this way the femoral head, if unstable, can be made to sublux. The procedure should also be performed on each hip separately, stabilizing the pelvis between the finger and thumb of the other hand. A clunk which is visible as well as palpable is elicited if the hip is dislocatable. This should not be confused with the click of crepitus which is commonly elicited and does not indicate any abnormality.

X-rays

(4) X-rays of the hips are less helpful in the neonatal period but later, at 3–4 months of age, the signs are more obvious owing to ossification of the femoral head. In high risk situations, such as a female breech, it is possible for the physical signs to be less than obvious but the X-ray findings quite conclusive.

Treatment

von Rosen splint

Plaster splint for late diagnosis

Splinting in abduction for up to 3 months is standard procedure. The von Rosen splint is commonly used but different orthopaedic centres have their own preferences. For the child diagnosed late, traction and abduction followed by plaster splinting in abduction are necessary. Some children may require an abductor tendonotomy in order to release the abductor spasm. Occasionally if abduction does not reduce the femoral head an open reduction is required. For the older child open reduction and osteotomy may be indicated.

Double nappies

Double nappies do not have any place except to temporize until an abduction splint is applied. It is important that all children with hips dysplasia should be under an orthopaedic

149

surgeon with a special interest in this problem since early diagnosis and correct management are most important for the child's future.

Painful hip

This is a common condition especially in boys and has many causes and these vary according to age.

Infancy, 0–1 year

Infection   Bacterial infection which may be blood-borne giving rise to a septic arthritis or osteomyelitis of the neck of the femur. Regrettably the outcome of this is poor since the articular cartilage is easily destroyed.

Toddler, 1–2 years

Infection
Rheumatoid
arthritis
Leukaemia

Infection still prevails but in addition juvenile rheumatoid arthritis and leukaemia can give rise to monarticular pain. A reactive anthropy following a minor viral upper respiratory infection can also occur but this subsides quite quickly with rest.

Children, 2–10 years

Traumatic
synovitis

Traumatic synovitis is the most common. In some cases the history is not always plain and so one feels that many cases ascribed to this might have other causes. Most resolve after a short period of rest.

Perthes
disease

Perthes disease, avascular necrosis of the femoral head, presents in a similar way. It, too, affects boys more than girls. As it requires longterm orthopaedic management all cases of painful hip therefore require careful scrutiny.

Tuberculosis

Tuberculosis of the hip is rare and because of this the diagnosis can be overlooked.

Adolescents

Slipped epiphysis can occur giving rise to either a painful hip or a painful knee owing to referred pain down the obturator nerve.

Talipes

There are many minor deformities of the foot found in infancy which correct spontaneously. At birth many babies feet are rotated medially. Most of these are positional deformities and show a full range of passive movement and require no treatment except passive manipulation.

Clubbed foot   Talipes equinovarus is the most common deformity giving rise to clubbed foot. It is important that this is strapped as soon as possible after birth and followed up by an orthopaedic surgeon, since often surgical orthopaedic measures are required. The association with congenital dislocation of the hip should not be forgotten.

Scoliosis

Although uncommon it is important to notice in childhood owing to its progressive nature. Once diagnosed the child should be referred to an orthopaedic surgeon, preferably one who has an interest in this condition.

12 Emergencies in paediatrics

Respiratory emergencies – Cardiac emergencies – Fits and coma – Metabolic emergencies – Gastro-intestinal emergencies – Genito-urinary emergencies – Miscellaneous emergencies

Advance telephone call to hospital in emergencies

There are certain conditions and circumstances where immediate action is required and where failure to respond promptly might jeopardize the child's survival or future health and development. When a child requires very urgent hospital treatment, a telephone call in advance to the hospital enables preparations to be made for the emergency to be dealt with immediately on arrival. There are some exceptional circumstances when it is reasonable to call an emergency ambulance even prior to seeing and examining the child, although in principle, this is not a practice to be encouraged.

Respiratory emergencies

Extreme urgency

Acute obstruction of the airway is one of the most dire emergencies where speed and appropriate action is essential.

Acute epiglottitis

Rapid deterioration

This is an infection giving rise to acute swelling of the epiglottis and vocal cords. Unlike croup, where respiratory distress is usually mild to moderate, respiratory obstruction can rapidly become severe. These children require immediate admission to hospital since they may well require intubation or tracheostomy.

153

Signs

(1) Sudden onset of fever, malaise and stridor in a child of the first decade in life.

(2) Increasing respiratory distress with subcostal, intercostal recession, sternal retraction and supraclavicular indrawing associated with flaring of the ali nasi. When the breath sounds are diminished in both lung fields, it is indicative of severe airway obstruction.

(3) The respiratory and cardiac rates are usually elevated but in the very ill child with severe hypoxia and metabolic acidosis they may be normal or low.

(4) Cyanosis.

(5) *The sweaty, grey, cyanosed child who is not struggling is in danger of respiratory arrest.*

Action

(1) Provided that the child is pink in air, rapid transfer to hospital should be accomplished without too much difficulty.

(2) In the child in extremis:

Oxygen

    (a) Oxygen is required by face mask.

Hydro-cortisone

    (b) Hydrocortisone intravenously may temporarily reduce oedema and improve the airway.

Sodium bicarbonate i.v.

    (c) Intravenous sodium bicarbonate, if available:

        (i) 5 mmol if the infant is under 5 kg,

        (ii) 10 mmol if the infant is 5–10 kg,

        (iii) 20 mmol for a child over 10 kg.

(3) If the airway is totally occluded:

Total airway occlusion

    (a) Insert a large bore needle or cannula through the cricoid cartilage and attach this to an oxygen line.

    (b) If a respiratory arrest occurs, *if experienced*, attempt to intubate with a small, firm endotracheal tube.

Examination of larynx contra-indicated

Unless the child is in imminent respiratory arrest, it is absolutely contra-indicated to attempt to look at the larynx. Inducing gagging in these children will invoke laryngeal spasm and precipitate a respiratory arrest.

Acute angioneurotic oedema

This can produce very rapid swelling of the face and neck. It often produces quite severe stridor but not to the degree of that caused by epiglottitis.

Action

(1) Intravenous hydrocortisone 100 mg will produce symptomatic relief within 4 hours.

(2) Subcutaneous adrenaline (1:1000) 0.01 ml/kg body weight given subcutaneously should produce prompt relief.

(3) Antihistamines are also effective.

Inhaled foreign body

It is not uncommon for children to choke.

Action

(1) Hold the child upside down and percuss the chest.

(2) Sudden compression of the abdominal viscera will often expel a foreign body from the lower respiratory tract.

Risk of pneumonia   It is important to remember that even if the foreign body appears to have been expelled some particles may have remained. In any case the respiratory tract has been traumatized and so the risk of a complicating pneumonia is significant. A

Chest X-ray   follow-up chest X-ray is therefore important.

Status asthmaticus

Early action to avoid status asthmaticus   In the management of asthma, therapy should be directed to avoiding status. If the asthma attacks are treated adequately from the beginning of an attack then status asthmaticus is relatively uncommon. Attacks which are treated late and inadequately are those that are prone to get into trouble. However, there are some children with labile asthma who very easily develop status in spite of all appropriate action.

    The child with moderately severe asthma will be pink in spite of being dyspnoeic and although showing considerable

Circumstances
for concern
and avoidance
of sedation

bronchospasm, the breath sounds in both lung fields are usually audibly good. The child who presents concern is one who becomes cyanosed, is grey and sweating and in whom, on auscultation, the breath sounds are significantly diminished. *On no account should such a patient be sedated.*

Action

Problems of
antispasmodic
drugs

All antispasmodic drugs can give cardiotoxic effects and should not be persisted with if cardiac arrhythmias are induced and also if no response is obtained to a standard dose. Do not give the same bronchodilator which has been given within the previous 4 hours.

Broncho-
dilators in use
Adrenaline

Among the bronchodilators commonly used are:

(1) Adrenaline 1 in 1000 given subcutaneously slowly on a dosage basis of 0.01 ml/kg bodyweight.

Aminophilline

(2) Aminophilline given intravenously slowly over a period of 10 minutes on a basis of 4 mg/kg bodyweight:

Aged 2 years   50 mg i.v.
Aged 5 years   75 mg i.v.
Aged 8 years 100 mg i.v.
Adolescent   250 mg i.v.

(3) Salbutamol can be given intravenously on a dosage basis of 5 μg/kg bodyweight.

Salbutamol
inhaler in
emergency

Salbutamol inhaler 1 puff (100 μg) can be given and repeated once in an emergency situation.

Salbutamol
given through
a nebulizer

Salbutamol given as Ventolin respiratory solution can be administered through a nebulizer and has greatly reduced the need for intravenous drugs in children with status asthmaticus admitted to hospital. It is given as 0.5 ml of a 0.5% solution diluted in 5 ml of normal saline administered through a nebulizer. While the hospital nebulizers are quite cumbersome pieces of equipment, there are current portable nebulizers on the market which many parents purchase for the purpose of giving nebulized salbutamol as well as disodium cromoglycate to their children. It may well be worthwhile considering such equipment in general practice to save the child the trauma of the intravenous or subcutaneous injection.

Terbutaline

(4) Terbutaline can be given much as salbutamol. Intravenously the dose is 0.01 mg/kg bodyweight to a maximum of 0.03 mg total.

A ventilator aerosol is also available made up in normal saline on a 1 in 100 dilution basis giving 100 μg/ml. The recommended dosages are:

Aged 3 years	weight 15 kg	2 mg terbutaline	
" 6 "	" 20 kg	4 mg	"
" 8 "	" 25 kg	5 mg	"
" 10 "	" 30 kg	6 mg	"

Oxygen

(5) Oxygen should be given to the child if it is cyanosed. If the colour improves it should still be remembered that there may well be significant airway obstruction and secondary metabolic acidosis i.e. beware that oxygen does not give a false sense of security.

Bronchiolitis

Respiratory syncitial virus

Clinical manifestations

This is severe airways obstruction of the terminal bronchiole due to the respiratory syncitial virus. Disease occurs in children under the age of 1 year and in many under the age of 6 months. The picture can be of increasing respiratory distress with hyperinflated lungs, high pitched inspiratory and expiratory rhonchi audible in both lung fields. While many cases of this disease will only produce moderately severe airways obstruction, there are some who can rapidly deteriorate.

Action

Oxygen

Aspiration of pharynx

(1) Moisture and oxygen will usually suffice to get the baby to hospital. It is important to aspirate the pharynx so that upper respiratory secretions are not adding further hazard.

Hydro-cortisone

(2) Hydrocortisone 50 mg given i.v. may help reduce bronchiolar oedema.

Salbutamol in emergency

(3) Bronchodilators have no place in relieving airway resistance under the age of 1 year but there are a few rare babies who do respond to salbutamol and in an emergency situation it is not unreasonable to try a stat. dose of 0.1 mg/kg bodyweight if the baby is over 9 months of age.

Pneumothorax

This is a rare occurrence outside hospital. It can occur in status asthmaticus and should always be considered if there is a dramatic deterioration in a child's condition. It can also occur in staphylococcal pneumonia giving rise to a pyopneumothorax. It should also be remembered in all cases of chest injury.

Action

Hospital admission
(1) Providing the child is fit enough to travel, he should be sent to hospital, receiving oxygen if necessary, where an intercostal drain can be inserted.

Insertion of needle into pleural cavity
(2) If there are signs of a tension pneumothorax and deterioration is rapid, a small syringe needle attached to a 20 ml syringe can be inserted in the pleural cavity and air let off until the child is fit to travel.

This should only be done in extreme circumstances as indiscriminate needling of the chest is not without its dangers.

Respiratory arrest

Immediate action
(1) Clear upper airway.

(2) Insert oral airway, hold the chin up and give oxygen with positive pressure with a mask and bag. *Attempts to intubate should only be made by someone experienced.*

(3) External cardiac massage will help ventilate as well as maintain cardiac output.

Cardiac emergencies

Severe cyanotic attacks

Tetralogy of Fallot
These can occur in tetralogy of Fallot. They seem less common these days since it is probable that most children with this condition are diagnosed and treated earlier.

Action

(1) Place the child in the prone knee/chest position.

(2) Morphine 0.1 mg/kg subcutaneously.

(3) Oxygen

If the child has frequent severe cyanotic spells he should be promptly referred back to the paediatric cardiologist for further assessment.

158

Emergencies in paediatrics

Cardiac arrest

Immediate action

(1) Clear upper airway.

(2) Maintain respiration by mouth-to-mouth breathing or with an airway and bag with oxygen.

(3) External cardiac massage.

(4) Intravenous sodium bicarbonate giving 20 mmol intravenously for an infant and 30–40 mmol for a child.

(5) Transfer to hospital immediately if there is any sign of response.

Cardiac arrhythmias

Digitalization

Heart block

Paroxysmal tachycardia is one of the most common. Although this may well respond to digitalization the child should be referred for assessment. Occasionally heart block occurs and this may be confused with fits, since it will produce syncopal attacks. Should a child remain unconscious with a heart rate less than 40/min intravenous isoprenaline (2–4 mg in 500 ml of dextrose solution) should be infused slowly until the heart rate picks up.

Congestive cardiac failure

Insidious onset in infants

Frusemide in severe cases

Usually this is insidious in infants, often with large ventricular septal defects and so antifailure treatment can usually be deferred until they reach hospital. Should the failure be severe enough to cause gross respiratory difficulties, frusemide can be given intramuscularly prior to transfer, the recommended dosages being:

Infants, 0–1 years   2 mg/kg
1–7 years   10 mg
7–10 years 20 mg

Fits and coma

Causes

Convulsions are common in children and have a wide range of causes from febrile fits, epilepsy, meningitis, metabolic disturbances, anoxia and cerebral injury. On diagnosing a seizure it is therefore important to realize the cause as this is often the crux of the treatment. While many children will have a fit and

Immediate
action

recover spontaneously, others will proceed into status epilepticus. Immediate action is therefore required to stop the fit and prevent anoxia causing brain damage.

Action

Cooling body

(1) In an infant or young child, where the initial cause could be a febrile fit, strip off the clothing and tepid sponge if the body temperature is above 39 °C.

Clear airway

(2) Clear the airway and keep the patient on his side and give oxygen if necessary.

Diabetes

(3) Should the patient have diabetes mellitus and hypoglycaemia, slowly infuse intravenous dextrose until the seizures cease and consciousness is regained. Alternatively 1 mg of glucagon can be given i.m.

Anti-
convulsants
Medication

(4) Anticonvulsants:

  (i) Paraldehyde 0.1 ml/kg i.m.,

  (ii) Diazepam given intravenously slowly:

    0–1 years 0.25 mg/kg
    1 year   2.5 mg
    5 years   5 mg
    10 years 10 mg

  The dose can be repeated if the seizure is not controlled.

Coma

All cases of unexplained coma require admission to hospital for investigation.

Meningitis

Fever and
neck stiffness

Lumbar
puncture

Any child with fever and any suspicion of neck stiffness requires admission to hospital for lumbar puncture. There are situations where meningismus arises from other causes but, even so, many of these situations require lumbar puncture in order to clarify the issue. When a child is difficult to examine and the physical signs are doubtful, then to re-examine 2 hours later is reasonable.

160

Head injury

Hospital
admission

All cases of head injury where a loss of consciousness was sustained, those cases with subsequent headache and vomiting and those which develop neurological signs all require admission to hospital.

Those cases in whom there is serious suspicion of intracranial or subdural bleeding require urgent transfer to a neurosurgical unit.

Metabolic emergencies

Diabetes mellitus

Diabetic ketoacidosis

This may present in either the previously undiagnosed patient or in an already known diabetic.

Newly
diagnosed
diabetics

Any child first diagnosed as having diabetes, whether with ketoacidosis or not, should be referred directly to hospital. Even when relatively well in the early symptomatic stages of the disease, they can rapidly develop ketoacidosis.

Known
diabetics with
mild
ketoacidosis

For the known diabetic, if the ketoacidosis is mild and the blood sugar is below 20 mmol/l, the insulin can be increased and fluids encouraged. When doing this it is best to increase the fast-acting insulin (Actrapid or soluble insulin) by 2, 4 or 8 units depending on the child's age and previous insulin requirements. It is important to diagnose the cause of the ketoacidosis which is usually due to infection.

More severe
ketoacidosis

Unless ketoacidosis is very mild, referral to hospital is necessary for stabilization. The child who is extremely ill with a blood sugar level of over 20 mmol/l could be given 4–8 units of short-acting insulin intramuscularly prior to transfer.

Hypoglycaemia

Dextrostix

From whatever cause this is potentially brain-damaging. Before treating it is ideal to confirm hypoglycaemia with a dextrostix reading.

The action to be taken is:

Immediate
treatment

(1) If the child is able to swallow, sweet drinks should suffice.

(2) For the unconscious child, intravenous dextrose given slowly until there is adequate response.

161

(3) If it is impossible to find a vein, 1 mg of glucagon intramuscularly or 100 mg of hydrocortisone intramuscularly can be given.

Adrenocortical crises

These can occur in children who have been on longterm corticosteroid therapy (including topical steroids) up to 2 years previously. It can also occur in those suffering from congenital adrenogenital hyperplasia.

Action

Child on longterm steroids

(1) A child known to have been on longterm steroids who suddenly collapses requires hydrocortisone intravenously immediately and referral to hospital for resuscitation and diagnosis of the precipitating cause.

Congenital adrenogenital syndrome

(2) Babies with congenital adrenogenital syndrome present with adrenocortical crisis at 2–3 weeks of life. They may present with vomiting, failure to thrive, hyperpigmentation and, in girls, pseudomasculinization. A firm diagnosis is urgently required and so prompt referral to hospital is necessary.

Hypothyroidism

Urgent blood sample

Avoidable cause of mental retardation

Any infant with any clinical suspicion of hypothyroidism should have blood taken for thyroid studies and it is important to stress on the form that an urgent result is required. If the diagnosis is proven it is best to refer to the local paediatrician for assessment and guidance on therapy. If diagnosed early enough it is one of the few avoidable causes of mental retardation.

Gastro-intestinal emergencies
Vomiting

The baby who vomits in the first few weeks of life deserves serious attention. Many such cases are feeding difficulties and babies that regurgitate but are otherwise healthy and gaining weight require nothing more than observation.

Pyloric stenosis

    Hypertrophic pyloric stenosis is always a diagnosis to consider, especially if the vomiting is convincingly projectile and there is failure to gain weight.

Action

Test feed

(1) Test feed – it is important to firstly aspirate the stomach and to measure the gastric residue following the previous feed and also for gastric lavage to be performed. Palpation of the tumour on feeding confirms the diagnosis of congenital hypertrophic pyloric stenosis. Referral for rehydration and correction of electrolyte imbalance is required prior to surgery.

(2) In the absence of palpating a pyloric tumour, in the non-thriving baby a diagnosis is still required and so admission to hospital may well be required.

Gastroenteritis

Diarrhoea with vomiting

Risk of dehydration

It is always important to remember that gastroenteritis is diarrhoea which may be accompanied by vomiting and that vomiting alone has other causes. *Babies and young children are very vulnerable to dehydration* with its associated electrolyte imbalance and so careful measures are required in these circumstances.

Action

Home management

(1) Mild diarrhoea with clinically less than 5% loss of fluid, no vomiting, warm hands and feet showing no peripheral circulatory failure, no hyperventilation and a good urinary output can be managed in the average good home. Provided the child tolerates clear fluids well and remains clinically well otherwise, conservative management should suffice. A glucose electrolyte mixture (Dioralyte) can be given and frequent small drinks advised. This regime should be continued for 24–48 hours until the diarrhoea abates, following which the child can be slowly regraded back to a normal diet.

Indications for admission to hospital

(2) *The child who deteriorates on the above regime, starts to vomit, has poor urinary output, requires immediate hospital admission and likewise the child who, at the onset, has more than 5% dehydration requires immediate admission to hospital for i.v. fluid therapy.*

Acute appendicitis

Any child in whom there is reasonable suspicion of acute appendicitis requires admission. Should the signs be doubtful it is reasonable to leave the child for 2 hours and then re-examine. Although acute appendicitis is rare under the age of 2 years, the morbidity and mortality are much higher, hence these children require more immediate referral.

Intussusception

'Redcurrant jelly' stools

Any infant or child with extreme colicky abdominal pain should be suspected of intussusception. As opposed to commonplace colic, the symptoms are more severe, they look ill, especially between bouts of colic and there may be vomiting. Rectal examination showing blood-stained stool (redcurrant jelly) makes the diagnosis highly probable. Prompt referral is therefore required since surgical exploration and reduction will be necessary.

Volvulus

This is uncommon but presents the picture of acute intestinal obstruction in the first year of life and therefore requires an immediate surgical opinion.

Hirschsprung's disease

This can present in the following circumstances:

Clinical features

(1) Neonatal with constipation, vomiting and abdominal distension. Rectal examination is followed by a characteristic gush of faeces and flatus.

(2) In neonates and infants toxic enterocolitis can occur with profound dehydration and shock.

(3) In the older child there may be a history of chronic constipation and abdominal distension dating from infancy.

Action

All cases suspected of being Hirschsprung's disease require immediate paediatric surgical diagnosis and assessment.

Genito-urinary emergencies

Wilm's tumour

Risk of delay

Any renal mass that is palpable requires immediate referral. It may be a Wilm's tumour, a neuroblastoma or a hydronephrosis. Delay in referral will only jeopardize the prognosis.

Urinary retention

Urological
investigation
This is rare in children and when it occurs there is a significant cause. These children therefore require referral for full urological and neurological investigation.

Acute renal failure

This, from whatever cause, requires immediate referral. Noting urinary output and blood pressure is important.

Paraphimosis

Lignocaine
and Hyalase
This is a distressing condition often leading to urinary retention. Injection of the oedematous ring with 1% lignocaine (plain) and Hyalase will often allow reduction of the paraphimosis some 5–10 minutes later.
Circumcision is indicated at a later date.

Torsion of the testis

Immediate
hospital
investigation
Any boy with clinical signs and symptoms to suggest torsion of the testis should be referred immediately for surgical exploration. If the testis is to be saved this should be done within 6–8 hours of the onset of symptoms.

Miscellaneous emergencies

Haematological

Causes
Severe anaemia and bleeding tendencies require immediate referral. Among the causes include blood loss from the gastrointestinal tract, haemolytic anaemia, leukaemia, idiopathic thrombocytopenic purpura, haemophilia and many other disorders. Establishing the diagnosis is vital.

Haemo-
philiacs
Many known haemophiliacs attend special haematological units. *When bleeding has occurred in haemophiliacs it is very important that immediate action is taken.*

Burns and scalds

Burns unit   Anything other than a trivial lesion requires admission to hospital. Severe burns and scalds are best referred to a burns unit.

Action

Analgesia   (1) Analgesia may be required if the child is in severe pain. Morphia or heroin can be used for the child aged 2 and over.

Saline or plasma   (2) In extensive burns an intravenous infusion with normal saline or plasma should be set up if the child has to travel a long distance.

Oxygen   (3) If the child has been involved in a fire he may have suffered pulmonary damage and anoxia or carbon dioxide poisoning. Keeping the upper airways clear and giving oxygen may be beneficial.

Cause   (4) It is important to try and ascertain the cause of the child's injury and the events leading up to it as this may well have medicolegal importance later.

Drowning

Many children of all ages drown each year. The outcome is influenced by the speed of action, whether there has been inhalation into the lungs or not and whether the drowning occurred in fresh or salt water. Many children die from hypoxia following reflex laryngeal spasm alone.

Action

Expel fluid   (1) On rescue compression on the chest with the face down to expel any fluid from the lungs or pharynx and aspiration of the pharynx is important.

Ventilation   (2) Insertion of an airway giving positive pressure with a bag and oxygen or mouth to mouth ventilation.

Cardiac massage   (3) External cardiac massage if the cardiac output is not satisfactory.

(4) Rapid transfer to a hospital with intensive care facilities including a ventilator.

Accidental poisoning

It is all too common for young children to ingest drugs, chemicals and any other noxious substances. The curious toddler who is exploring his environment will try anything that is left around.

Action

History   (1) First, establish the substance and the amount thought to have been taken and the time at which it was taken.

Vomiting   (2) If the child is fully conscious it is important to induce vomiting (*except if it is known that the child has ingested a corrosive substance or paraffin*). Vomiting can be induced by sticking one's fingers down the back of the child's throat and if this does not induce vomiting tinc. ipecacuanha paediatric emetic draught 10–15 ml followed by 1–2 glasses of water will usually induce vomiting and this dose can be repeated after 15 minutes. If this is not effective, gastric lavage must be done.

Unconscious child   (3) In the unconscious child it is important to see the airway is clear and that the child is not hypoxic. Gastric lavage should only be performed with a trained anaesthetist at hand.

Hospital referral   (4) All cases should be referred to hospital, since although in most instances the ingestion is trivial, in others the amount is considerably greater than the history indicated.

Intentional drug overdoses

Psychiatric assessment   This occurs usually in adolescent children and these require admission to hospital for their own safety. Psychiatric assessment of these situations is important since many of these children come from disturbed and unhappy backgrounds.

Non-accidental injury

Any new case or new episode of child abuse requires immediate investigation.

Action

Hospital admission   (1) The child can be admitted to hospital and most paediatric units will instantly accept such a child. The hospital

167

social workers can then assess the situation and convene a case conference and hopefully appropriate action can be taken.

'Place of Safety Order'

(2) Alternatively contact local social services who could, if necessary, apply for a Place of Safety Order from a magistrate and the child can be taken to either a local paediatric unit or to a foster or children's home. This order lasts up to 28 days.

(3) Contact the police who can issue a Place of Safety Order immediately which lasts up to 7 days.

Discretion

Cases of child abuse cause anguish to all those involved. It is important not to unduly delay action for the safety and well being of the child, but when evidence is on suspicion and not established fact the utmost discretion must be exercised.

Psychological problems

Child guidance clinic

While many of these can be referred for routine assessment at the local child guidance clinic, there are some instances when it is reasonable to ask for admission to a paediatric unit. These instances include the following:

Perpetually screaming baby

(1) The perpetually screaming baby. There are many aspects to this problem but whatever the underlying cause, parents get to the point of being beyond control when denied sleep for long periods. An admission to hospital affords them an opportunity to revive themselves and also for the overall problem to be evaluated.

(2) The child with gross behaviour difficulties.

(3) The very unhappy child.

Index

Problems in Paediatrics

Vallergan forte   113
vasovagal attacks   66
varicocele   131
Velactin   37
Ventolin   156
ventricular septal defect   72–3
vesico-ureteric reflux   49–51
virus infection   24–8, 54, 150
   and diabetes   85
vision testing   121–22
vitamins   16, 18, 19, 57, *see also*
      named vitamins

walking reflex   120
warfarin   18
   and breast feeding   16
weaning   18
weight, birth   117
weight gain in babies   16, 21
weight measurement   113
Wilmer's tumour   131
Wilm's tumour   51, 164
Wysobee   37

X-ray   28, 42, 49, 70, 71, 102,
      103, 144, 149, *see also* chest
      X-ray